S.T.R.O

The Ultimate Blueprint To

Penetration Orgasms

By Montique Stephon

CONTENTS

PREFACE v

LOVING ONE'S SELF 1

I CAN'T USE MY PENIS 7

BAD PENIS EFFECTS 13

SOLUTION: RITES OF PASSAGE 23

ERASING PORN DAMAGE (A WORD TO THE MEN) 33

ABOUT ME 49

THE HIPS DON'T LIE 57

TRAINING STROKE SKILLS 63

RHYTHM MOVEMENT & THE OCEAN 81

RHYTHM TRAINING 87

SEXUAL GEOMETRY 93

POSITIONS ARE AUTOMATIC ANGLES 101

SHERLOCKING 112

KNOW THY SELF 119

THE AUTO ANGLE 123

WE JUST HAVE TO CHANGE THE WAY WE THINK 129

FOCUS VS FORCE	133
SEXUAL RECALIBRATION	139
HURRY UP AND BANG	149
YOUR END IS HER BEGINNING	153
EXIT STROKING	157
STROKE FREQUENCY	159
INFLECTION & MISDIRECTION	163
STUTTER STROKING	167
RAW GUY TALK; SIT INTO YOUR STROKE	171
REVERBERATION STROKING	177
WOMEN THAT ARE SHOOK ABOUT CONFIDENCE	181
LACK OF CONSISTENCY	193
THE BEST FOOD STROKES	199
CONCLUSION : WHAT WILL YOU LEAVE HERE?	205

PREFACE

As a man, it's extremely important to understand the value of self-worth. You must embrace your worth in order to be an attentive father, cherished husband and vigilant protector. Fail to recognize this, and you will never effectively transfer that type of confidence into any sense of security for loved ones. Owning your value is different from the way we love and appreciate things we buy. It adds a sense of calm to the way we love and appreciate our successes.

Such self-assurance guards us from holding too tightly onto any possession as a means to validate ourselves. This appreciation is resistant to fads and addiction to retail. It is as timeless as a lion watching his hard-won pride play within his territory. It keeps us directly connected to who we are, what we represent and our passion and courage to change the world for the better.

This book is a testament to the importance of men recognizing their own self-worth and their own self-value. After all, the male sexual identity has been thrown under the bus as of late thanks to apologetic 'yes men' who placate for female support. This is the case specifically because of the fact that we as men do not recognize our own sexual power, and by sexual power I'm not speaking about forcing sex upon someone. I'm not speaking about using our wealth or status to attract anyone in hopes of 'getting any' either. I am speaking on the importance that we as men recognize ourselves as sexually powerful due to our unique abilities and capacities. My goal is to speak to those of us who want to be appreciated for who we are and what we have instead of being compared to others. Those of us who feel this way must recognize that this appreciation comes from inside of ourselves.

My hope is that in reading this book you recognize that there is a way to develop this power within yourself. The keyword is 'develop,' which means that it's not going to happen by osmosis. It's something that you must constantly improve upon so that you as an individual are able to own it and so that it can never be taken away from you; anything that comes easy and without any type of struggle can erode and dissipate in the fashion. My work as a speaker has been fruitful for one reason and one reason only: that healing others with these issues I am healing myself. The reason for this is because in this society we are constantly comparing ourselves, we are constantly sizing ourselves up against other men, we are constantly downing our own potential and our own successes because of others. I too suffer from this. This book is my contribution to trying to assert and find a solution. I hope that some of the things that you learn within this book help you to recognize yourselves as powerful and to make you unafraid to become so much better so many ways.

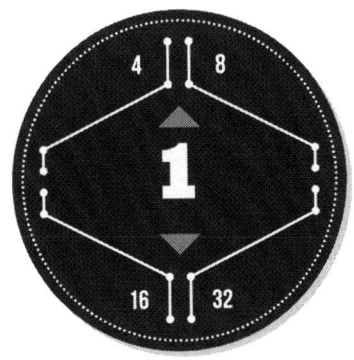

LOVING ONE'S SELF

If you do not love yourself, well, you cannot do anything well, that's my philosophy. - Nawal El Saadawi

Many of us wake up in the morning to a life of someone prescribed to us. We follow a system of models that gives us direction and dictates what is to be our destiny. This is the process of putting on masks others might say is the cost of 'doing business' if we want to be successful.

The problem is that this understanding carries over into all areas of our lives. That's when it becomes dangerous and detrimental to our health. It's one thing to fall in step with a certain behavior or protocol in order to follow standards set by a person paying you to perform a particular job. It's completely different when you impose someone else's standards on yourself wholesale. The inability to take off this mask, the inability to disrobe this outfit that we put on in order to succeed within our careers can seduce us into losing who we are. In losing who we are, we lose touch with our natural abilities. We use lose touch with what we bring to the table that makes us unique and without the innate understanding that comes with being an original, you can never grow. Millions upon millions of men will never come to understand the power that they truly have because they suffer under dozens of layers of masks to satisfy their bosses, family and the women in their lives. In time, authenticity becomes revolutionary.

It all starts with recognizing and appreciating the man in the mirror. This all starts with loving oneself, loving one's body and loving one's uniqueness. These three things are inextricably linked and tied together; when you love your body and you can look in the mirror and you can appreciate the different attributes that your unique body has you are ultimately telling yourself that you love yourself. This is made possible because these are attributes you have been born with, elements you ultimately cannot change. These are genes that have been birthed into you as an individual. When you understand the love and appreciation that you have for your body is directly connected to the love and appreciation that you have for self, something revolutionary and magical happens. It's truly the key to unlocking one's purpose.

This is why the ancient Egyptians said that "knowledge itself was thing that all of us to strive for as our main goal while living on this planet." Knowledge itself is like a flower; once it blossoms open we're able to see our true purpose that takes us to another plane when it comes to the potential. We are introduced to our ultimate potential realized. It emboldens us and makes us more confident than ever. The society we live in makes it extremely difficult to do. Commercialism is inextricably tied to inadequacy. If you are content and confident in who you are, you are not in the market for being sold anything. There is no need for the latest diet, car or phone.

Appreciating yourself to this degree will perpetually refresh and renew the thoughts about losses and failures, victories and successes in positive ways, reinvigorating your approach every situation. Every situation can then help you to become a better you and closer and closer to being who you want to be.

 Carlton Davenport I thought initially, that this was a set of useful external exercises for sexual strokes and ab development as a secondary benefit.. There is so much more of a benefit as far as emotional, confidence, and radiating and renewing sexual energy.
Yesterday at 5:47pm · Unlike · 👍 2

Now that Raúl had finally broken up with Alexi, the plan, he knew the plan his uncles and father had for him to recover would be to get blitzed at bars and run through an impressively long string of women. That ridiculous, "what-the-fuck-was-I-going-through?" sex where forgettable women agree to getting thrashed behind clubs, in friend's houses and in gas station bathrooms.

That was the way guys got over a woman narcissistic enough to constantly to try to cheat her way into a better situation with someone else. A good guy getting shitted on always called for going into beast mode.

Uncle Hector brought one over to Raúl's apartment as Raúl sat on the couch in the dark one Thursday night to watch the Spartacus series on Netflix. Hector turned on the living room light. "What the hell are you doin', bro?"

Raúl could tell from the volume that Hector had been drinking. Raúl quickly wiped his eyes and sniffled. "Chillin', man."

Hector looked over to the flat screen then motioned for someone to come in behind him. She did, and hung onto his arm for balance. She was bleary-eyed off alcohol and held up a lilac halter top with the slightest of ease. Raúl figured she couldn't have been no more than 23. Such smooth, golden skin. Her big, curly black hair, five-inch wedges and tight jeans set off tremors in Raúl's loins.

"This here is Salma, bro. I told her about you and everything."

Salma stumbled against Hector's shoulder. She scratched her hair and smiled at Raúl. Hector nudged her toward him. "Go meet my nephew, girl."

Raúl smirked. It did seem stupid to be only 29 years old and done with the world. But something told him better. To not sweat it.

"It's cool meeting you, Alex – " Raúl groaned.

Hector grimaced, "See?" He pointed Salma to hurry to him. "You see? My bro' is hurting. That bitch messed him up. Suck his dick or something."

Both Salma and Raúl burst out laughing.

"Wow." Salma plopped onto the couch. "You kinda totally fuckin' pushy, Hector, y'know?"

Hector shrugged his shoulders; "Yo' my friend's in hell, girl. Fuckin' help him."

Raúl reached out to Salma. "It's been cool meeting you."

Hector waved. "Aaargh! No, bro'!"

Raúl smiled. "I just –"

"No, she might suck it. You never know –"

"Hector are you mental?" Salma yelled. She through her tiny hands up in the air. "I'm in the room hearin' you, okay?!"

Raúl motioned her closer to him. Salma scooted her tight hips closer, her head wobbling ever so slightly. Raúl whispered a request in her ear, her hair tickling his face. Just as he took in the smoke and perfume on her neck, she got to her feet and staggered around the corner into his room.

Hector gave Raúl the thumbs up. "Damn straight up, man. Thought you was gonna pussy up on me, bro."

Salma returned hanging close to the wall holding Raúl's tanned bed spread. With a surprising sense of grace, she steadied herself to gently cover him with it. Hector tilted his head like a puppy hearing a new sound. Salma kissed Raúl on his forehead, flopped down next to him like a nerd's book bag and picked his cell phone up off the table in front of him.

MONTIQUE STEPHON

"This is my number." Her voice went sweet and easy. *"Okay?"*

Raúl nodded and turned to Hector. "Thanks, really. I need my time though, Hector. I'm good."

Hector froze. Salma slid over, reached for, and grabbed, Hector's hand. She pulled herself up, held Hector's large face between her hands and gave him the most solid look of confidence she could: He knows who he is, what he needs. That's very rare. Leave him be.

Salma turned off the light. They left, leaving Raúl to contemplate rest, jacking off to Kanye West's 808 Heartbreak album, screaming himself hoarse into his pillow and, ever so quietly, working this stroke skill program he had purchased through Paypal for some confidence.

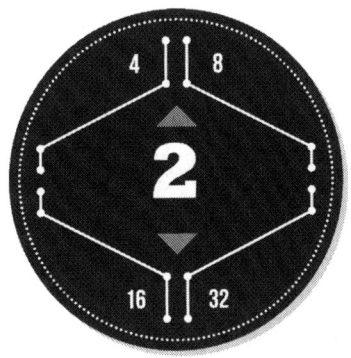

I CAN'T USE MY PENIS

Happiness comes from the full understanding of your own being.
- Marina Abramovic

There is a simple truth that a majority of men don't want to address, a simple fact that situates itself as being a huge decision-maker around the things that we do. It affects things that we don't do, the aspirations that we move toward, the women that we choose and the life that we choose. It's likely the smallest but the biggest thing in our entire lives and that is our penises. A man's connection and appreciation for his penis is likely one of the things that has the most control over how he feels about himself. Yes, it's truly unfortunate, that in today's society a majority of men are unhappy with their penises, upwardly about 85% of men in United States are unhappy about their penises.

I wonder how many of that 85% actually know a reason that they should be happy. In our society there's only one way and that is through actual measurement. In many cases the way that a man feels about the size of his penis is the only thing that he has to love about his penis, so if that individual is not sized in a way that would make him comparable to what he feels women want, he ends up having a negative relationship with his penis. Through that he creates a negative sense of self-worth and that's something that reverberates through his whole life.

A man's love for his own penis makes a lot of sense; the penis is the only body parts that actually has a key role in bringing life into this world. A man's penis plays an important role in the way that men pleasure women as well, so how can a man effectively have good relationship with themselves or a partner if he does not have good relationship with his penis?

The fundamental flaw lies in the fact that our society doesn't offer more reasons and ways for men to appreciate themselves beyond measuring one's size. In many cases men with larger penises actually have less successful sex lives, women that married men with large penises get more divorces than those that don't per capita. These statistics show that is possible to have a member that is actually large by conventional standards and still fail at pleasing a woman. Therefore, if a person feels momentarily like they value themselves in that respect, that value can drop immediately following a session where that individual is not able to perform effectively.

We as men are uncertain about how to use our penises and thus require Band-Aids like feeling good about our size to cover lack of understanding. Out of a hundred men, 99.999% of those men have only given women orgasms by accident. We keep a 'one style fits all' mentality using one penetration in and out style technique with different women. As a group men lean on the use of positions in order to denote their sexual prowess. However, is shown that if a man is not able to adequately engage a woman from one position, chances are they will not be able to satisfy her from a different position.

The default is to depend upon luck and pray for a miracle, but there is far more available to us than that. We have an ability to understand exactly how to master the use of our penises, we have the ability to recognize the benefits of such knowledge no matter which way we are cut. No matter which way we are shaped there is something that is beneficial to each and every one of our penises. Each of us can encapsulate various different styles in various different techniques that are connected to our unique bodies and unique penises. This makes each and every sexual experience that we have unique. This gives us the ability to appreciate our bodies because we recognize our capacities as being special. We recognize our contribution to sex as being special. We know that we can give unique sensations that no one else could duplicate because they are coming from us in our most natural state.

If we do not build the means to activate these powers within ourselves we will stay uncertain. We will stay insecure and our actions will compensate for that uncertainty. We will find ourselves doing things to protect our egos. We will find ourselves hurting people in order to protect our sense of self. We will find ourselves connecting with individuals who we know that we can dominate specifically so that we feel good and safe about our abilities. There is the temptation to construct false realities in order to help maintain a belief in something one is inherently unsure about. This leads to injuring not just ourselves but loved ones and our society.

• • •

Tom hated the saying as soon as it came up on the screen: "There is love in freedom." He scooted back from his computer screen, yawned and stretched as if he were trying to reclaim the full space of his shitty cubicle. Shitty indeed, he thought as he glanced over at the stack of hard drives in the left corner and overflowing garbage can to the right. Shitty he thought, yes, but it was his. All his.

He looked at the picture of him and his girlfriend Sasha. It was a picture of them in the park on a sunny day, her kneeled down in front of him on the grass and him behind her with an arm around her, gently pinning the back of her neck and head against his barreled chest.

Sasha smiled at the camera. Or was it something else? Her right hand rested in the crook of his arm, as if ready to try to peel his arm loose should he decide to choke her. The hand reminded him of his tantrums in public of this and that guy looking at her. Of returning home in a quiet boil until he slid his way into her and pile-drived himself to an orgasm. He thought of that meaty thump as he collided with her, how it sounded as if the air was being knocked out of her. Part of him knew good and well she endured it as opposed to enjoying it. Maybe the force of it impressed her enough to keep her respecting him. A pang of guilt riddled his chest; what a dumb thing to say. All because of fear. He thought of how it was not her at all, but the fear that overtook him of guys that appeared sane with a full head of hair crossing their path.

Tom closed his eyes and clasped his fingers behind his head. Christ... Sasha used to think it was cute when he puffed up at guys over her when they were at the bars and malls. Now, not so much. Not at all now, really. How could Sasha not want to leave if things were easy enough for to do so? Tom sighed. He looked back at the picture. No, he realized, Sasha was not smiling. She was squinting in the sun while keeping her man's love from cinching into slow but gradual a chokehold.

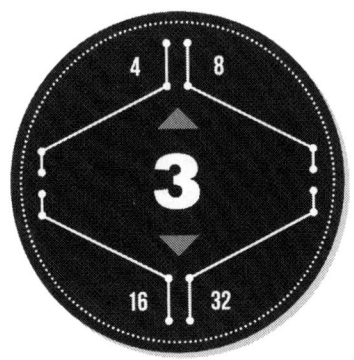

BAD PENIS EFFECTS

The evil that is in the world almost always comes of ignorance, and good intentions may do as much harm as malevolence if they lack understanding. - Albert Camus

When men are unable to grasp the way to use their penises, bad things happen. They become overwhelmed with uncertainty and fear. Billionaire and financial wizard Warren Buffett once stated that when we as individuals know what we are doing, there is no fear.

Consequently, when men talk about being afraid to ejaculate too fast or nervous about performance or how to satisfy a woman, there lies the basis of many peculiar habits and attitudes that ultimately damage one's quality of life. Men not understanding how to adequately use their individual penises is the cause for all male self-confidence problems. I hold it responsible all of the systems and things created for men to maintain egos and fortify self-confidence.

Not knowing how to use your penis is similar to not knowing yourself. Not knowing how to connect to your body's natural abilities to please a woman sets you up for failure not just in your relationship but in your ascension as a man because you lack the ability to stand on your own and know that in and of yourself you are sufficient.

This lack of appreciation and lack of understanding for oneself has reared its head and some truly ugly systems across the globe. A perfect example is the Machismo culture prevalent in Spanish-speaking countries. It is also prevalent in Portuguese speaking countries like Brazil and Cape Verde.

Machismo culture finds its strength and its purpose in the idea that men should actually own women. To that effect many might say that the idea that a guy being protective does not mean that he owns them because in the Machismo culture the argument is that men are merely protecting the women in their lives. However, studies show that within Machismo culture there are some the highest incidences of spousal abuse and domestic violence to date. There has not been much research done on the considerable mental abuse that takes place in the Machismo- based cultural relationships. I predict that the numbers are truly astronomical (The culture is deeply entrenched in Latin culture and because of the fact that it's been around so long there are millions of people that actually appreciate and enjoy the Machismo culture that are actually women).

The truth of the matter is that within these cultures, there is actually a fear of women progressing themselves. There is actually a fear of women being sexually expressive. Now why would you think that there would be a fear of both women progressing themselves and women being sexually expressive? The answer lies in both of those cases women have the ability to discover what good sex is, and men are unconfident and uncertain about how to provide it. Much of Machismo culture is based in this whole concept of the male leading and to be honest I don't really feel a problem with that so much as the notions and practices that come along with it. It ultimately leads to those who created Machismo culture truly not being confident in how to operate and use their penises as individuals.

Machismo culture keeps an unnatural hold on to the idea that women should have sex or be engaged prior to dealing with the specific man and woman. This is because an individual who does not have confidence within himself and appreciation for his body and the knowledge of how to use his penis is literally afraid that they will not be able to stand up and perform as well as other men. They become afraid of becoming exposed. They don't want her to know that he is inadequate with his tool, so they would rather her be very inexperienced and not be able to tell the difference between a man who has mastered the ability to please a woman using his unique body and one who knows nothing about what he sees in adult films.

Machismo aside, this has been an issue that has plagued civilization for centuries - the lack of confidence that men have in themselves and in their abilities. It reverberates and actually has changed the way men engage women due to the fear that they are recognizing that there are options when it comes to man's abilities in bed. Rather than develop his own capacity to please a woman masterfully, he would block her from knowing that mastery exists. That is the power of denial, the power of uncertainty and the power of fear.

Another way that this problem manifests is in the development of the male psyche through the ugly system of genital mutilation. Many look at cultures that perform genital mutilation and try to connect it to cultural background, religion, and historic beliefs that have gone back centuries but there's one thing that's very common in it all: sexually unsatisfied women.

Sexually satisfied women don't exist in these cultures, and that's because the cultures in and of themselves have become so afraid of being chastised for their performance that they cut off the ability for women to feel pleasure altogether by removing parts of their bodies that would actually give them pleasure. This is not connected to religion; this is connected to male ego because as men, the only time that we want to relieve a woman of feeling pleasure is if we are afraid of the pleasure that somebody else gives her is better than the pleasure that we could give her.

You have to ask yourself, who wants to be in a relationship with a woman you could not please? No one! So rather than learn how to please woman and learn how to use your body masterfully in order to please, communities around the world opt to mutilate the genitals of the woman instead. Fear can drive men do horrendous things.

A less violent (and actually more consistent and pervasive) way that the uncertainty and lack of confidence that we have in our penises can be found in relationships when men cheat. There are tons of books on cheating - and there are tons of reasons why people cheat - but one of the key reasons why men cheat that no one examines is the need for accreditation. Many people might say that it's in men's nature to cheat. Many people might say that it is natural for men to want to spread seed in many women.

Polygamy and polyamory is something that's been around since the dawn of time. One thing that stands out that makes what goes on today so much more harmful (than anything that could have been within a polyamorous relationship) is the fact that men in our time try to convince women that they have feelings for them when they don't, in order to gauge an authentic response to the sexual abilities. Men don't want to do it with prostitutes, night workers or call girls. They want to deal with real women with real emotions, and they want to deal with them because subconsciously they want to test the potency of their thrusts.

In short, they want to know if they still have it. They're uncertain about the means that they have as it pertains to sexual prowess. They use these women to confirm their talents. They require an emotional component so that they can tell if the woman would allow herself to truly feel and be swayed by their sexual capacities.

This wreaks havoc in the life of that woman when she finds out later that the individual is married and that everything said to them was a lie.

It creates a cycle of abuse that trickles down from them into their sons, with whom they treat with an increased amount of anger and criticism. It continues on to future suitors who they hold in less esteem because of the fact that they were injured by a man who basically wanted to use them as a crash test dummy. When a man doesn't know himself for certain, fear is ever present, looking over his shoulder, telling him that he needs to know *for sure*. This is why these individuals have a very hard time staying in a committed relationship. This is the reason why these individuals have to engage with many women, keeping them in the dark. It is so that these men can feel good about their abilities.

It never dawns on them that if they were to train and develop their abilities with a healthy and mature mindset from the beginning, they would prevent broken relationships, damaged children, bruised egos and very disgruntled angry and unsatisfied women. Ultimately, they're never able to truly appreciate the benefits of a monogamous relationship. Many don't think about the fact that when monogamous, one has the most access to understanding their mate. It offers true communication with them because of the fact that we have the most direct experience with them. We have the opportunity to learn them and turn that information into pleasure when we make love.

Monogamous relationships are amazing for self-discovery as well, because that person being so open to you enables you to recognize new things and new abilities that you possess. When you don't have an understanding of the ways that you as an individual move best when it comes to sex, it damages the capacity to grow.

A foundation of understanding is needed in order to build upon it. Foundations allow you to develop new abilities that build and stack on other abilities that you have. This has an important role when it comes to monogamous relationships, because of the fact that your partner will change. It is up to you to understand how to adapt your style to take their change in stride. Their changing is part of being human, but just because they may want different sensations doesn't mean they don't want you. They want you, most likely to see if you can modify yourself and the engagement to meet their new pleasure.

In many situations where I've seen a confident man be able to 'answer the call' of such changes, they were actually able to find the silver lining to it all. This included new realms of pleasure pertaining to the sexual relationship because nothing changes in a vacuum. Everything changes 360°.

She requires a new type of feeling to feel pleasure, a new type of intensity, a different style. Fine. You can give her that and show them how you can adapt to them. They adapt to you, and this is not just in the bedroom. It reveals itself in the communications in your daily life, it reveals itself in the way that they will be able to go out on a limb for you and take chances when it comes to you, and because you've proven yourself you find yourself receiving more positive support.

When women are truly satiated, they show their appreciation via reciprocity across the spectrum of your relationship, not just the bedroom. You can see it on multiple levels across location, time and space. Men have an essential need to learn to appreciate their bodies and unique sexual abilities. It is extremely important that men recognize their sexual self-worth because if they don't, history shows us the result.

・・・

Mark struggled with the thought as he swirled around inside Paige's milky thighs, searching for traction. He recalled so many pornos of skinny, limber girls taking monster penises with expressions no more intense than if they were taking a dump. He had hoped this wasn't the case with Paige, that she was different. After all, she was so cute and silly with this eternal ponytail of black hair, the one girl he liked pairing up with for assignments at culinary school. But no, she just had to be the proverbial hallway to his Tic Tac (Tac: echo). He stroked slowly, listening for any kind of a response from her. Hoping.

Paige closed her slanted brown eyes and inhaled, slightly. Mark's nostrils flared. The thought... it crept up higher in his spine until it tickled the back of his brain. <u>I got tricked. Only a whore could be this huge</u>. He could feel that pounding in his ears and sense his vision starting to go cloudy. <u>Did she fuck the whole class or something? Fuck!</u> He slammed into her and began to replay some of the worst things he had ever heard women say at such a moment: That's all of it? Just finish. All the laughter from girls as far back as the fourth grade left some cavern in his heart like a wave of bats and swirled up into a black cloud behind his green eyes. If she exhaled one decibel too loudly, with some kind of a tone to it, it would guarantee the other girls she hung out with at the culinary school would hear about it. Mark shook his head and slammed into her heart-shaven mound.

So then this is what it's going to come to, he reasoned. And why not beat her to it? Why not have some sense of power by being the one to at least initiate the decline? Say she and her grand canyon of a cunt sucks before she says he does. He sensed tension in her and slammed in again, a thought came to him.

What was that stroking program? Ah! The Egyptian strokes program, designed to give her a feeling of girth. Mark sighed and quickly shifted to an inverted missionary position, turning counter clockwise so that his right leg was outside of Paige's. And then, Mark timidly started the Egyptian Hip Slide, dropping a deep, scooping lift stroke at her center. He then slid his hip off of her left hip for increased torque and pressure. Paige gasped. Mark pulled his shoulders back, she felt it.

Once he was off to the side of her hip, stretching it just enough for some respect, he came with another lift stroke from that angle.

Paige looked into his eyes, then down to his hips and smiled. She gripped his hip. "Oh," she laughed nervously, "what's that?"

Mark's mouth went dry. He brought it back over her hips and sent another solid pump to her center. And then slid it off her hip again. For another angled pump, primed with torque against her left lips and right wall. She bit her pierced bottom lip and lifted her hips to meet his.

"This, well, in Egypt --"

"Keep, just keep doing it."

Suddenly, the campaign he had hatched as a backup plan should the sex go wrong, vanished. The hatred, ready to attack her for men he could only imagine her for having, evaporated. He no longer feared her hole, or any woman's hole, for he was whole.

Mark continued, feeling her walls contract against the base of his rod, thanks to the angle. Paige let her head sink into the pillow. Her hand slid from his hip to his ass. Ah, he thought, all the awesome conversations they had about comic books and being gourmet chefs that built up to this could remain in his heart. She no longer was the whore from which he had to protect his psyche. No, now she was just as he had seen her, a different kind of emo chick. Now, he would not fall in step with bitter, intimidated men she suffered through. No, things were different – because he was different.

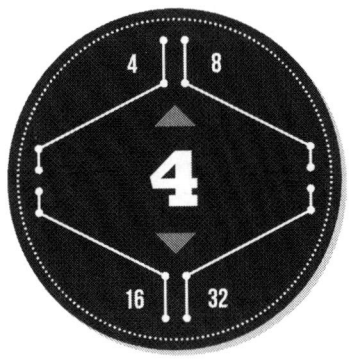

SOLUTION: RITES OF PASSAGE

Rituals, anthropologists will tell us, are about transformation.
- Abraham Verghese

The importance of men knowing themselves and appreciating their sexual prowess is the floorboard of his confidence and floorboard of his ego. If this confidence is not instilled at a formative stage, a tendency to use other people, social constructs and material things in order to compensate. This means a renewed vision for rites of passage.

Cultural rites of passage in many countries across the world have a process where young men are guided into manhood by the older fathers, brothers, cousins and community members. Knowledge and understanding is passed down so that young men find the means to understand themselves to recognize themselves. In each of these cultures there is a process where the young man is held to going off by himself and developing himself. This is after the men in the communities surround him and give him the tools that he needs to chisel out his own identity as a man. This process allows young men to benefit from the extended and connected knowledge of the men that have gone before him. He's not having to step in the same potholes make the same mistakes as those who have gone before him, so each generation becomes better and better because each generation filters itself so that the generation following it makes fewer mistakes. So what happens when such markers are taken away?

Today, such rites of passage are almost extinct. Boys lack clear markers on their journey to becoming a man. If you ask them when the transition occurs, you will get a variety of answers: "When you get a car," "When you graduate from college," "When you get a real job," "When you lose your virginity," "When you get married, "When you have a kid," and so on. The problem with many of these traditional rites of passage is that they have been put off farther and farther in a young man's life. 50 years ago, the average age an American man started a family was 22. Today, men (for ill or good) are getting married and having kids later in life. With these traditional rites of passage increasingly being delayed, many men are left feeling stuck between boyhood and manhood. College? Fewer men are graduating. And many that do "boomerang" back home again, spending another few years figuring out what the next step in their life should be. As traditional rites of passage have become fuzzier, young men are plagued with a sense of being adrift.[1]

---

1 http://www.artofmanliness.com/2008/11/09/coming-of-age-the-importance-of-male-rites-of-passage/

Western culture is devoid of all rites of passage. Young men grow up in the world making the same mistakes over and over and don't have the means to ask questions. They don't have an opportunity for people to educate them about things that they would not come to know except through experience. When it comes specifically to sexual experience (and learning from experience) this can be detrimental simply because they are engaging in an act that involves someone else's emotions and also has the potential to bring a life into the world. If there was a means to bringing rites of passage back as a prominent part of the male experience, we would see an end to genital mutilation and the Machismo culture.

We would see the fear that men have and the unrelenting self-criticism that they bear down on themselves dissipate. We would watch them learn to appreciate the process that they themselves invested in when making love. When being intimate with a woman they would begin to appreciate the changes that women go through versus being afraid of them because they would have an ability to adapt.

Men wouldn't feel as though if a woman changes and her interest change that there's no more interest in him. They wouldn't feel the need to go and engage other women (or lie to and take advantage of other women) in order to test out sexual capabilities. He would have a healthy sexual self-worth and value. He would not need to look outside of himself or relationship. Many males go through a process where they feel an affinity for women who lack a certain amount of independence and lack a certain amount of financial stability, a certain amount of education because they are fearful that those women would not find them attractive otherwise. This based on a man who does not appreciate his own sexual self-worth.

A man has to see himself as being more than the car that he drives, or the income that he generates, or the connections that he has. He must look at himself as a healer and warrior, an individual who has the capacity to satisfy a woman mentally and do so with such expertise that he has no equal. This man has developed his own style and has been able to apply the knowledge of self intimately to extend into his woman. He is able to deconstruct a woman's thinking. He doesn't require other people to congratulate him or to hoist him up in order for him to feel sexually powerful. He knows he is sexually powerful and walks in that power every single day.

When acknowledging this power, such a man ceases to use the weak tactics of the over-intoxication of alcohol or date rape drugs to trick women to sleep with him:

Some 15 percent of women are raped while incapacitated from alcohol or other drug use during their freshman year at college, according to new research. The report, published in the Nov. issue of the *Journal of Studies on Alcohol and Drugs*, also helps to offer a clearer idea of which college freshmen are at particular risk of what's known as 'incapacitated rape.'

Researchers found that freshmen women who'd been victims of such assaults before college were at substantial risk of being victimized again. Overall, nearly 18 percent of students said they'd been raped while incapacitated before college, and 41 percent of those young women were raped again while incapacitated during their freshman year.

The students' views on alcohol also seemed to be involved. Young women who said they believed alcohol can enhance a person's sexual experience were at increased risk of incapacitated rape during their first year of college -- regardless of whether they'd been victims in the past.[2]

Please consider that these are the statistics for an educated population of young men, men with no rites of passage. This shows a growing culture in the younger generation in the music of drugs being the same type of shortcut they experience at the click of a button in social media. Drugs to shortcut the feeling of boredom, fear and the possible pain of rejection. A proper rites of passage program will show them how to relax and socialize, so they know how to let the flow of good conversation allow a woman to become comfortable enough to do what she will with them. He cherishes a fully lucid woman that is simply high off of being near him, so much so that she stares him in the eyes as she bites her bottom lip and slides out of her thong. More than anything, a young man who has gone through the proper rites of passage program will see himself too worthy to resort to such a pathetic state to get a woman to have sex with him. That kind of confidence alone can be seen as cocky enough to attract women on its own merit.

---

2 Journal of Studies on Alcohol and Drugs. "Study finds high prevalence of incapacitated rape among college women." ScienceDaily. ScienceDaily, 18 November 2015. <www.sciencedaily.com/releases/2015/11/151118070751.htm>.

One crucial element that must be added to the rites of passage process is the solution to the fractures in the male ego. Elders in our community (and the men who are older than us) have shared experiences that will teach us numerous things about the world, about communication, about being a man - but there needs to be this component that speaks specifically to sexuality, to male sexuality, and the means of understanding one's body and the sexual power that it holds.

We need to learn how to appreciate our bodies; we need to learn how to appreciate our penises. We need to learn how to find the sexual superpowers hidden in our bodies. We need to be able to find effective means to use our penises with the bodies that we have for the greatest effect so that we should never want to be anyone else. The power that we have and the unique the abilities that we possess make us special and allow us to give a gift that only we can give.

When this takes place and this installment is added to the rites of passage concept, what will happen is that instead of men belittling one another because of the bodies that they have or because of the penises that they have or because of the things that they lack in general, we will see men to start helping one another by sharing tricks and tactics. They will give each other ideas and things methodologies that worked for them. We will see the sexual sciences grow by leaps and bounds because it will become a community of knowledge sharing as opposed to community based on secrecy, degradation and chastisement. The solution for us is the resurgence of rites of passage within our society. The key component that needs to be connected to the rites of passage deals with something that we call the stroke, something gravely compromised by pornography.

• • •

A new age nutcase. That's how 38 year-old Jerome's uptight, conservative family saw him. At the same time, none of them admitted to the fact that they sent an awful lot of their problems his way to figure out. "It's like you're that touchy-feely sex intimacy couple in Meet the Fockers" announced Roslyn, his sister who called one Thursday night to warn him that Freddie, her sexually stunted, 21-year old son (his nephew), was on his way to his doorstep. "Talk to him. It's girlfriend problems. Charles only says so much to him."

The doorbell rang right the end of her words. "He's here," said Jerome. "Talk to you later." From what Jerome could make out of the situation, Freddie was not well endowed. He remembers taking the boy to the indoor pool at 17 and the boy shifting and turning at odd angles in getting out of the pool. Freddie almost passed out when Jerome lead him to the locker room to shower up and change clothes. Now the kid had a girlfriend and, thanks to his antisocial dad and over protective mother, the kid's self-esteem over it was probably wrecking his social life.

Jerome knew the routine: let Freddie peruse his library collection in the living room until he hit a book title that so weird, but that Freddie could not help inquiring about. That would be the opening to get at whatever the issue was with him. Sure enough, Freddie's lanky frame *stopped at the Kama Sutra book. Jerome feigned ignorance, focusing on his binge watching of Game of Thrones from the living room couch. Freddie adjusted his skinny jeans.* "That smell, what that again?"

"That incense is Nag Champa," *Jerome sipped from his cup of chamomile tea.*

Freddie nodded and pulled the Kama Sutra book from the bookshelf. "So this all about Eastern sex positions or something?"

"India to be exact. They say it was created by woman who were tired of not getting pleasure from men doing the same tired movements," *Jerome shot a look over to Freddie to gauge his attentiveness,* "so they created the positions so even the tiniest, most inexperienced guy could take care of business."

Freddie looked back and nodded thoughtfully. "You use this stuff or you just keep it out here to get hippie women wondering?"

Jerome smiled and sipped. "Both, and all kinds of women."

Freddie flipped through the book. He began to mumble his words. "Doesn't really say what to do if you just, y'know, finish too fast."

Jerome studied his face turned away toward the bookshelf, what he saw of it. "A lot of that comes from men overthinking the moment out of lack of confidence, of men not confident in their skills."

Freddie scratched the back of his neck. "Yeah, but not everybody has like, a baby arm or whatever."

"Don't need one. If you have skills whatever you have is enough."

Freddie turned around completely. He tugged at an earlobe.

Jerome put Games of Thrones on pause. "First off, most guys think of the actual motion with only the head of their rods in mind. The real work comes in on the sides of it, where it feels like a ribbed condom."

Freddie chuckled and shook his head.

"Think about it, the head is the most sensitive, so you wind up in some female you've obsessed over to the point that you're ready to burst just processing the fact that you got this close to her."

Freddie snorted and sat down on the lounge chair with the book in his lap. "The sides of the dick though?"

"That's what engages her walls. It's all about her walls." Jerome sipped more tea. "I had a girlfriend in college when I was about your age. She had run through enough of her share, but she was so aggressive with me I didn't have time to doubt myself and be scared."

Jerome began to recall her. Those tight black shorts. Volleyball playing girls were amazing. "She was on top at all these weird angles. I was like, is she trying to rip my dick out my body?"

Freddie laughed out. His cell phone began to ring. He ignored it.

"I am not Mr. Baby Arm, but she slept like a baby afterwards." Jerome laughed at that one, even though it was her own doing. "I figured it out, the angles thing and tried her again in about an hour from an angle I thought up in my head, one with one leg forward so I curved to the opposite direction inside her. Same thing."

Now Freddie looked as if he was envisioning something. "The sides of your dick."

"Yeah, hitting her sides."

Freddie's phone rang again. He looked at it. Jerome could tell it was Freddie's girlfriend, the bossy one that probably was taking too many liberties with him because his low self- esteem.

Freddie smirked at the screen. I got something for you. He then shook his head and looked at Jerome as if to say, 'why was such a revelation so hard to come by?'

Jerome smiled. "The world's got a lot to learn, dude. And our family's part of it."

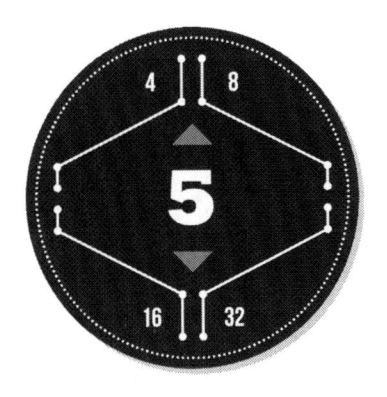

ERASING PORN DAMAGE (A WORD TO THE MEN)

Some habits of ineffectiveness are rooted in our social conditioning toward quick-fix, short-term thinking. - Stephen Covey

A lot of us have the ability to see a movement and just duplicate it, do you know how we got that ability? We developed that ability friend watching adults in order to learn how to walk. It progressed when we grew older at play, mimicking idols and friends. This is a gift and a curse though. It's a gift because now you know that you can tap into something that will allow you to learn and allows you to build muscle memory. It's a curse because of looking at the wrong things has us subconsciously copying what is incorrect and can ruin you from the inside out. I'm talking about adult film, pornography.

How many adult film clips have we men seen? I've seen may be a couple thousand if not more. Each and every one features guys hammering a woman's vagina. When I was watching it I was unknowingly creating muscle memory . I was subconsciously I'm absorbing that this is the way I'm supposed to do it, I was learning from it, it looks real enough right?! The lady is laying there getting it. She's screaming. She's sweaty. She's enjoying it and what he is doing? He is throwing it into her hard, fast and strong every single time. So in my mind I'm thinking that this is what I'm supposed to do. When I go home to my lady it's what I'm going to subconsciously use what I learned from the porn as a frame of reference. I expect the same things that seemed to work in the pornos to work with my wife or girlfriend. But in reality what you are doing is hurting her, numbing her vagina and also causing her to link sex to fear and pain. It can take away her ability to orgasm because instead of allowing herself to feel the pleasure from sex, she braces herself for pain. they are hurting her. Many of the things that we pickup from porn could actually tear her vagina and I know a lot of you have done that. I have, too. I'm not proud of it.

The thrusts that you see on TV is for TV, for cameras. Directors know how to get angles that really make you want to pull your meat out and jerk off. That's their intent, to titillate you, excite you. They know how to get angles and have the people stroking to turn their hips in certain ways so that you can see more penetration. It's how they pick the positions and how they pick the way that he's going to plunge into her and pull out of her. All of that is pre-scripted and has nothing to do with what feels good to her and has nothing to do with what was good to him. It's about giving the camera what the camera needs!

I want you check this concept out really closely; if you have watched at least three or four thousand different porn clips and it's been etched into your brain, how do you get rid of that, how do you erase that from your muscle memory? Your subconscious has read this information. This part of your mind operates when you're not paying attention to it and what times do we least pay attention to our mind? Yeah, during sex so, so it's happening is even if you don't want to hurt her even if you don't want these things to happen, this part of your mind is taking over. Because your body learned this material, because your body absorbed it and because you've done it every time that you have sex, you have a theoretical and physical connections to this programming. The only way to undo it is if you replace it with something else. Until that is done, many will find themselves with "dirt roads" plowed through their brains according to an informative article in Relevant Magazine:

Every time a person views porn, or eventually even thinks about porn, the burst of dopamine strengthens the connections between cells. The stronger the connection, the easier it becomes for cells to communicate on that path. This idea of the brain changing itself is called neuroplasticity. Whether learning to ski, learning to speak a foreign language, or looking at porn, the more we use a particular neuropathway, the more our brain changes, making the pathway stronger.

These neuropathways are like footpaths across a field of waist-high grass. Walking across the field when the grass is so high requires significant effort. But each time you walk along the path, it gets easier.

The grass gets trampled, worn down, and eventually becomes a dirt path.

Someone who doesn't watch porn, or is not yet addicted, has yet to develop sensitized "weed-whacked" pathways. But the porn neuropathways of someone whose brain is addicted are weed-whacked and trampled down so that they have become the path of least resistance. Porn becomes the path of least resistance in the brain. And the easier the path, the more likely we are to take it, even when we don't want to. The creation of this path of least resistance is called sensitization.[3]

We are adopting moves from guys we think are great but in reality on camera they do it for about five or six minutes. What happens then is they change the camera angle, lighting and position of the cameras. He can be there beating his meat from anywhere between 15 and 20 minutes while the whole set changes are going down. He then goes into the position and starts fucking over again. Yeah, those long strokes where he's really pounded it like that? No cat is going to be doing it like that for 15, 20, 40 minutes straight bro, they're not doing it like that, these guys are having hydration breaks on top of that.

These women they're smashing a lot of times are going to be in situations where their vaginas are turned off. This dude is having sex with dead space and that is how come he can do all this crazy shit with his cock and she won't even budge. She is just taking it because she has Ambesol in her. Do you know what Ambesol is? It's the stuff that

---

[3] http://www.relevantmagazine.com/life/whole-life/features/29332-this-is-your-brain-on-porn#rrjzCvACVOX3f3Si.99

you put in your mouth when you get you tooth pulled it; makes your whole face numb.

Additionally, have you ever seen how porn actors put their hands on their hip, you ever wonder why they do that? Oh, you thought they were doing that because is somehow helping the stroke or putting extra juice on their strokes right! Nope, it has nothing to do with that the director tells them to do that so their hand isn't in the way and you can see the action, you understand what I'm saying?

The director is telling these dude how to screw! When you guys are mimicking these porn guys when the majority of them are being told what to do by a skinny, no sex having sucker director trying to catch all the penetration on camera. That the reason why I didn't do anything other than in and out strokes back then. You know what the in and out stroke is?

Yeah, you do. It's the only one that you know how to do. That's the one where you push all the way out and push it all the way in. So what if I told you doing so you're actually pulling all that lubrication, all that juice out every time you stroke like that? You're bringing it into the air where it dissipates. That means that it dissolves or dries up. You're pulling all the juice out of her and putting your cock back into her dry. No wonder she's all beat up. There's the tearing, the bleeding. She complains that it hurts. The reason why is because you are doing it to her like she is one of these porn chicks and she's not numbed up with Ambesol.

What's more, you're not juicing her up with lube every five or six minutes like they do in porn. They couldn't have sex with the women in the pornos like they do if they did not have the woman fully lubricated and numbed up. That's right.

So what you are going to do is keep your strokes tight. That means you're not going to pull all the way out every time you start a new stroke. You're only going to pull all the way out after she is thoroughly lubricated and come all over you because then when you're pulling out and that moisture is coming out with you, you know she has a whole ocean waiting back for you that's going to make sure that she gets right. It's going to make sure her vagina doesn't tear and it also going to make sure that you don't get all chafed up. A lot of you wind up with cuts and whatnot because you are not thinking about your stroke. Time to upgrade, don't you think?

• • •

As Dante finished the first 80 strokes of the 80-10-10 on Aisha's clit, he could tell she was more talk than anything when it came to sex. Either that or she simply had come across too many dudes in Timberlands who bent her over, grabbed her braids and lost their minds at the sight of her healthy and bouncing, pecan-colored ass.

The wannabe row-house thug type that figured some tongue-kissing and spitting on their dicks was enough to get going. The type that figured the more they were about just getting it in, the more 'hood and manly they were. She did not realize she was now on Howard University's campus, dealing with some educated dick.

S.T.R.O.K.E

So, then, apparently, she thought he was kidding when he told her he would start with 80 strokes across her lips and clit with fingers, tongue, the head... Either way, 80 damn strokes. 80 of them shits.

As they lay in his dorm room bed, she grabbed his wrist just as he finished slow-dragging the underside of his head over her glistening, raised clit. She inhaled restlessly and tried shift to sit him up in her. He complied, only 3 inches in... so that he could tease her with the 10 mid way strokes.

"Alright, boy. Come on."

Aisha ran her hand over the waves in Dante's low cut hair and tried to flip him over to get on top. Dante cackled. Hell to the no. Ain't about to get on top and rush though to a full-on fuck. Naw, Aisha. Not here.

Dante gave Aisha the ten midway strokes with strict adherence to the 3-inch range. He even pulled a move he had studied in his psychology class by wrapping his hips with the blue bed sheets to hide his penis from her sight. Aisha licked her thick lips and looked down during the strokes. She whimpered at the sight of the covers. She looked up at Dante. You playin' right? There's more dick, right? After the ten mid strokes, he dropped the full situation into her, even pushing off with his toes. She gripped his triceps, closed her hazel eyes and shook her head like a fat kid eating the first mouthful of a piece of cake. "Mmmm! Shhhhit."

Dante let it sit deep to enjoy her quivering along his length. He remembered how she responded to the underside of his head coming down over her clit like a light switch being flicked off. Ah, that same sensation came from the drop stroke. He commenced to dropping it, lifting his hips above hers, setting them onto her butterfly tattooed lower belly and dragging them down under hips.

Aisha hissed and licked her lips. She pulled the cover away and shifted to allow enough space to see their slick and heated piston and pump agreement. Dante watched her eyes, how they looked down and then up into his.

"You ain't gonna watch it long stroke in and out?"

Dante shook his head. "I ain't on no corny porn shit, don't need to see it like that. I see mines every day. I wanna see you."

Something changed in Aisha's energy. The tough, street-talking exterior fell to the side of the bed. He could see it in her softening face.

She sat up on her elbows and kissed him as if she meant to bring life into his body. Dante played in her braids and gradually, went back to the drop stroke.

Between the crackle of the cheap mattress, a wet gurgling began. A wet, thankful sloshing. She moaned and hissed, timing it to block out the sound. Dante stopped and whispered across her hairline:

"Shh, I wanna hear it talk."

He put another stroke in. She laughed nervously just as the sounds of wetness started up again.

"Stop Aisha, I can't hear it."

She obeyed and he stroked. And it sang.

"You like that for real?"

"Who don't like the sound of a pussy that wet?" Dante kissed her eyelids. "Good pussy sound like stirring mac and cheese."

Aisha laughed, "You stupid."

Dante continued with the drop stroke, staying tight to her, to which she bit his bicep as if he were truly made of chocolate. "You all up my clit wit' it, wit that stroke."

Dante made her pull back her shaved mound with her fingers for better contact with her clit and then continued. She rolled her eyes. Hot damn! This motherfucker right here... He put a finger over her trembling mouth.

"Let it talk."

Aisha's stomach began to quiver and jump. "Ooo, goddamn you playin' wit me."

Dante sped up, almost setting his hips onto her with a clap.

Aisha whipped her head from side to side. "Keep fuckin' around, hear?"

Dante suddenly switched to a drop/lift combo stroke, which rubbed his hilt against her clit and mound with a surgical accuracy. Her gurgling did not stand a chance to be heard over her own pleading. Aisha closed her eyes and buried her face into his chest. "Oo, shhhit please keep fuckin' around."

Dante continued. Every stroke became a turning of a page of the book of her life of sensuality. He kept stroking until he got to a blank page. When he did, he started pushing off with her toes. Staying close. Keeping the wetness going, making the pages stick with gratitude.

He could tell she was close. Time for some reverse psychology:

"Hold up, did I say you could come?

Did I say you could come?"

Aisha howled and shook her head. "Don't say that! Don't–" Her mouth formed a perfect O. He sped up, hammering stroking the butterfly tattoos on her quivering belly to jump like popcorn. "Oh, God!" Aisha writhed under him, coming in hard, wet convulsions. "Shiiiiiiit!"

Dante switched back to his drop stroke as she whimpered through the aftershocks. Aisha, glassy-eyed and clawing up his back, howled again. She then went quiet, letting her wet grip kiss, suck and pucker at his manhood.

She wiped her face. "Another plate of mac and cheese?"

Dante nodded to let her know that he was man known to go for seconds.

The World Is Baby Stroking

Growing up, I just wanted to be like everyone else. I didn't value or understand the beauty in being different at the time in my life. - Marisol Nichols

It's really difficult doing things that are different. It's very difficult to actually participate in activities that nobody else that you know is participating in. It's really easy to really fall in line with the rest of society and just tell yourself, 'yeah, I don't need to work out my sex game. I've got that naturally.' It's really easy to tell yourself that you're good with what you have, with absolutely no investment in it. Think about it. How good would you speak, how good would you play ball, how good would you be at your job? Could you even add or subtract? Could you even talk, better yet, if you actually did not practice?

So right now, a lot of y'all are still on some 'gaga goo goo' when it comes to your sex game, simply because you have never learned to put words together. You've never worked at it. Imagine if you did. Think about the difference between the way you speak now and the way you spoke as a child, as a baby, before you understood vowels, before you understood consonants. Think about the different ways you were able to communicate when you started to actually work at it, when your mom and dad started talking to you on a regular basis and started correcting you and giving you more words to add. Bro, that's no different than what I'm doing. I'm talking to you. When you get on that ground and you knock these strokes out, you are practicing, just like when you practice speaking. You're using the terms, you're using the terms, you're using the nouns, you understand? You're just using them in a different context. You're exercising your game. In the end, you have to realize that when you're at the point when you're about to make love to a woman, and you're standing in that mirror, you're in the bathroom, and you're in the mirror, you catch a glimpse of yourself, you know that at that point in time, there's something you can say to yourself to remind yourself just how much work you have put into your sex game. Reminding yourself that you have a better chance at making this woman orgasm and giving her the most pleasure that she's ever felt than anyone that she's ever been with before. Why? Because you work at yours. Does that make sense?

The first person you're supposed to turn up before making love is you. So you go in that bathroom and you look in that mirror and you tell yourself that she's about to get the work. 'I'm about to give her an experience that she's never, ever had before. That she will never, ever have again.' And it'll be the truth. I mean, I tell guys all the time, shit, log into the website, check the app, speak to other guys like yourself and ask them have they ever dealt with a woman like this before.

Give everybody her dimensions. Tell them the type of personality that she has and get feedback. Because see, when you go in with a plan, when you go in with strokes, ideas, concepts that have worked with similar styles of women, you can rotate those different ideas, those different strokes, those different concepts until you find her specific combination, until you find the perfect combination for her. See, that's what we're here for as your community. We want you to win. We want you to be the best you can be with her. You tell her 'yeah, I work on my stroke game' and she at that point knows that we're the best in the world. We are the best in the world when it comes to penetration, when it comes to sex. We are the best just because of the fact that we train to be the best. We put work into our stroke. We have value. You understand that? We have value. We have something that matters.' Or you can say nothing and just blow her mind on the sly.

Before you make love to a woman, get in that mirror and stand in your power. You are not getting pussy. You are not getting chocha. You are not getting pussetta. You are blessing her with some A-level quality penis. Some A-level quality cock. You are blessing her. And you're going to get in that mirror and tell yourself she deserves it, she's done this, she's done this, she's done this. 'I'm going to let her have it tonight and I'm going to leave her remembering me. I'm going to make her feel and understand that I appreciate her.'

• • •

It came to Vic at 6:12 a.m. just as Dee slid from her side to her knees, raising her ass to him and flattening her chest across the mattress; the patent doggy position where he always lost it. She motioned for him to get after her with her right hand as if telling some kid to bring her the remote. Vic grabbed her hips and thought of that, by remote. Dee was church mouse quiet through the whole thing and now, instead of telling him to "do it" (come and finish, which he had grown to resent), she simply flipped into the position that gave the same result. She was going through sex, especially in the morning like this, on auto-pilot.

Vic almost lost his erection at the thought. The excuses to keep quiet because of the kids didn't cut it, all of the sudden. And so, with heated focus, he put to use this Stroke Skill idea of his penis being a paddle instead of a poolstick. He entered slowly, then smiled at himself from the revelation. A modification that the housepainter could truly grasp. My dick is a paintbrush!

Vic's typical stabbing stroke changed instantly. He moved in and out with a fluidity that made it seem as if he was under water. The meanstemmed paintbrush brushed walls thoroughly with a lift stroke. Yes, he remembered, that's what it was called. Dee looked back as his hips became his wrist. When he pressed in to the hilt, he snarled at the wicked idea of pushing off with his toes for more pressure. He did so and pressed her hips into him to truly send a message. Dee groaned like she was being worked over on a massage table. He pulled back and re-entered again with the same push-off with his toes. Dee groaned again, then hissed. He shook his head, today was starting off quiet well for the new DaVinci of Dick.

As he exited, he caught her shivering. Her hips then began to press up against him. He continued painting her walls a new coat of ecstasy.

Dee eventually hissed and lifted up so that she stood on her knees. She reached back over her shoulder to cradle the back of his head. "What you doin'?"

Vic quietly took her by the back of her neck and guided her back down, face down, into the mattress. "Wakin' you up."

She whimpered. He continued passed 6:42 a.m. The sun slowly took over the horizon to add definition to Dee handfuls of the sheets. Vic continued with the pushing off of the toes. "What's that breakfast gonna be like, huh?"

"Eggs and bacon, baby."

Vic stopped just before withdrawing to feel her clutch and quiver at his penis. "None of that lame Cinnamon Toast Crunch?" Vic slammed in for impact stroke.

Dee squealed, hissed and smacked the mattress. She lifted herself up so her breasts swayed. "Oo! Eggs and bacon, baby."

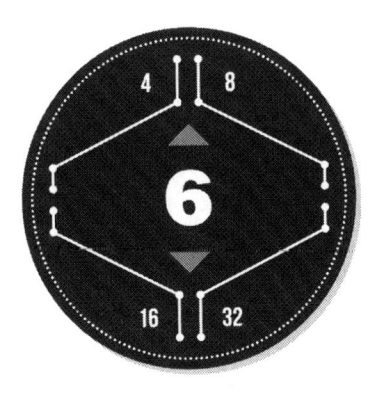

ABOUT ME

An understanding of the natural world and what's in it is a source of not only a great curiosity but great fulfillment.
- David Attenborough

I dealt with very low points in my life. My success in redefining my body and my confidence in myself is the reason I am here today. It took the tragedy of almost losing my entire livelihood and a very close friend to start studying the S.T.R.O.K.E. (systematic tactile rhythmically organized kinetic exercise).

I want to tell you how it came to be so that we have a connection and mutual understanding. Tom Matheke Fischer is an amazing guy, a lawyer and accountant in the early 90s. He made a fortune trading commodities on Wall Street. Unlike a lot of other successful people Tom did not forget his roots and when he made it big he offered to help build the MMA Training Facility we had talked about in college (We were huge fans of the UFC and SHOOTO very early on).

With my connections in the fight world and Tom's finance background, we were up and running in no time and right in time as the MMA interest started booming. It was going so well that we were attracting many of the best teachers around at that point. I bought a house and Tom bought more homes.

It was about a year or so in when Tom came into the gym and told me he was dropping his business interests in the gym and moving back home. It was his wife. She apparently was medicated for depression and Tom felt he was at fault because of her inablity to climax and thus feel sexy.

I was overwhelmed. First of all, we had never discussed Mary (his wife) and definitely not in this capacity. But, he was my friend and business partner and the foundation for our business was his knowledge of how to engage investors...this problem quickly became my problem.

Supposedly, Tom, had at one point and time been in marital bliss complete with great sex, intimacy and a really satisfied wife. However, over time what she liked seemed to change and what Tom knew no longer worked. She stopped having orgasms and soon after stopped wanting to have sex and there after fell into a deep depression.

Tom had cajoled her into visiting a therapist and discovered that she could not even bring herself to orgasm felt incapable of receiving pleasure. The psychologist suggested medication and a warning to

Tom "you must solve this or you will lose her." At this point my friend was almost in tears and as uncomfortable as it was seeing this huge guy break down, I tried to focus on how we might find a solution. After convincing Tom to give me some time to find a replacement for him, I set about the task of uncovering a way to have Tom stay and that meant figuring out a way to reunite he and his wife. I hated that I was in this situation. I was a fitness trainer for fighters. I was not some marriage counselor but I decided I would work through the process with him and together we would have to succeed, my life and his depended on it.

I transferred my classes to another instructor and virtually lived in the library for days on end. After ruminating on the problem for days, I boiled the whole situation down to the base problem. In the past Tom and Mary had a great sex life but then something happened, something changed. I researched this and actually found that a declining and unfulfilling sex life was the #2 reason for divorce.

Apparently, when this happens everyone takes it personally. The guy thinks something is wrong with her and she thinks something is wrong with him so it can quickly escalate into infidelity or divorce because people want a second opinion a confirmation that it is not their problem. It didn't seem so complicated to me, I figured if their bodies changed, you simply would start with what you knew they liked and then just experiment from there. I learned that he knew very little about what she liked. I mean he knew the stuff all guys know, touch her here or this position, but nothing around the details and specifics of what she liked sexually. And when I thought about it, neither did I. I was perplexed. After more digging I would come across an article that would change everything. Tucked away at the Library at the National Institutes of Health was an article on something called the Coital Alignment Technique or C.A.T. It was a way of aligning your self with her to help her achieve orgasm through sex.

Again I called Tom ready to burst but he said had tried it and after seeing the diagram I sent to his phone said that is how she USED to like it... well he said some unkind things. I could tell he was starting to move past the phase of sadness into the phase of anger. I needed to move faster. The C.A.T was the best thing I had found at the N.I.H Library. I talked to a friend who was into Chi Kung Kung Fu who told me about Mantak Chia and Tantra. Chia defined Tantric Sex as the capacity to use energy transference through breath this would increase blood flow and stamina. Their research showed that a Dr. Shin, a Chinese doctor of sexual healing, recorded a very interesting position that had similarities to the C.A.T but was different.

The C.A.T was in a missionary-like position. Dr. Shin's was with her sitting on top. The similarities were in the motion and the positioning in their intimate parts. I recognized the importance of the positioning in regards to the clitoris, the in stroke, friction and exit. A light bulb went off in my head. If the C.A.T worked at one point, what about trying different kinds of C.A.T movements at different rhythms?

One was sure to work. The Coital Alignment Technique was not a position, it was truly a technique one that could be used in many ways, Dr. Lin had proven that with his eastern version. I went home and looked at several hours of video specifically of women bringing themselves to orgasm. I clocked approximately 13 ways they moved their hands and moved the toy inside them. With each one they did a variation of Coital Alignment.

I was a little wacked out by the time I got back to the gym. The guys had already closed everything up for the day. I felt determined though, I was a creative coach that came up with dozens of training sequences to throw kicks and punches from several different angles. I knew I could transfer it over to something else. I took out my note pad and started crafting movements that would recreate each of those 12 different sequences I had recorded from the internet. Picking up my pad I saw my scribblings from the Tantra breathing chapter of Chia's book. I breathed using the instructions I had noted and suddenly each movement I made seemed to charge me for the next one. I turned on my camera. With Tom and me both off in space, we had completely forgotten about an inspection that our gym was due. When we found out that the inspection had taken place, we knew we were in trouble.

A court summons came in the mail, they were looking to close us down for a series of outstanding fire code violations. We were told we would need to do file what seemed like an ocean of paperwork within the next several days. Tom looked less like a Yale Graduate and more like a bewildered court-appointed attorney. He was looking bad. All I could think of was how is this guy going to get motivated enough to handle that stack of papers because I damn sure don't know what to do with it. We stopped at the gym and I told Tom to hit the shower and come out ready to train.

I wheeled the TV into the training space and along with my notes; I showed the video outlining how each movement implements Coital Alignment and what it effectively does to her. The first day we got through 3 and we had drawn a crowd at the gym. All chuckles aside everyone had to admit…it made sense. We all looked like a cheerleading squad the way we rah rah rah'd for him on his way out. My phone was ringing off the hook that night with several of the bros from the gym raving about having tried the stuff out with their girlfriends, but I had to catch them on the answering machine because I was busy with mine. Tom, the one that I was waiting to hear from, didn't call. He didn't turn up the next day either. I called his phone several times and sent emails.

I was worried I was planning for the worst when I popped up at his house in Bethesda, Maryland a couple days later. I started to leave after knocking a couple times thinking he wasn't there, but then I heard a couple thumps and Tom comes stumbling out in a robe. Before I could say anything he starts hugging me like we won the Super Bowl.

He was beaming, I heard Mary yell downstairs, "Tom what are you doing down there?"

He smiled and we shook hands then he scampered back inside as I headed back to the car.

We took care of the court situation Tom was on top of work like never before and I was back to normal kicking guys in the head for hours at a time a day.

One thing had changed, everyday those of us who were around for what had become known as "Operation Stroke" met up a couple times a week after class for 15 minutes or so and do this special set of exercises. The way they empower your whole being and make you incredibly strong are only seconds to what they do with your lady.

Tom is currently off doing business in China now but even today we check in with each other and our extended family of bros around the world to make sure we are doing our workouts daily. Men, your world will change because your perspective about yourself, sex, and intimacy will have changed drastically for the better. With your new skills you will enjoy the challenge of pleasing woman, putting value on what you bring to the table. Your abilities will be a point of pride with you. You will love yourself and you will appreciate what you bring to the bedroom and to a relationship and that will only improve as you continue to build up your skills. When you feel that way about yourself it leads to orgasms that will be earth shattering for you both.

The Zenity vision is can be your guidelines for your new perspective and skills. Great sex has nothing to do with your size, or with money or power. It comes from understanding yourself and your body.

When you practice the base moves you can then begin to improvise, adding more and more into your arsenal, creating your own style to fit your body type and your rhythm.

Replace your old view of sex and the male ego with Stroke Skills's vision and it will bring success, vision, ambition, style, and skill into your life. You will find pride in your skills. Women will value you for your skills, they will look at you and wonder what you bring to the table and you will be able to show them

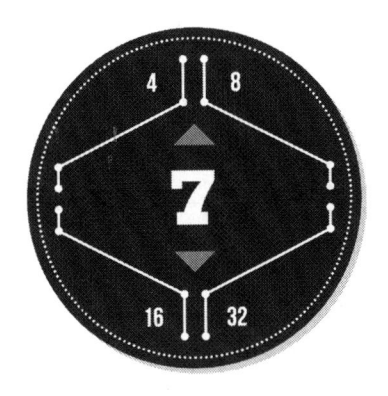

THE HIPS DON'T LIE

I make music for the hips, not the head. - Norman Cook

Yes, pool sticking is addictive. It's addictive because it's the only stroke that we've ever seen in our life. It's the only stroke that we find to be masculine. It's the only stroke that we've seen work for the most part. Why? Because we watch a lot of TV. We've seen that stuff in porn since we were kids, and as we grew up, we stroked many chicks that way and we thought that they liked it. So that's why we kept doing it. In reality, as stated before, pool sticking hollows a woman out, dries her out, makes her insensitive and if you've had any other strokes, it'll make those strokes less effective because of the fact that you've numbed her vagina. You can imagine what pool sticking is, right? That's when you push it straight in, and pull it straight back out. I can't lie. I revert back to pool sticking on a regular basis. But I've come up with something to help me stay on point.

What you do is you want to keep your eyes focused on her hips. You don't want to stare at just her hips, because then she'll think you're not finding her attractive. So you have to alternate between looking at her, into her eyes and looking at her hips, but the thing is, if you can look at her hips, you can almost kind of make a practice out of using the stroke that best works with the way that she rotates her hips. Very few women are going to stay there and stay still when you're stroking. They're going to be moving their hips up and down, they're going to be moving their hips left to right, in circles, etc. And you, you can think about it like, how do I match a stroke to the way that her hips are moving? Just keeping that in your mind. Keeping that as something to do. It's almost like a reminder that you should not stop stroking and that you, of course, not go back to pool sticking.

When you start applying strokes based upon the way that her hips are moving, she really gets into it and you see a defining difference between that and how she acts when you're just doing your in and out pool sticking, rabbit strokes. I know that that shit looks cool. I know that it's normal. I know that when we think about being men and we think about putting it down, that's the action that comes to mind. But in reality, that's just the action that comes to mind because of TV, all those jokers that you thought could stroke, they really can't. They've got 1 or 2 strokes, maybe. Maybe. And that's sad.

. . .

S.T.R.O.K.E

Jacques made a point of keeping the lights on with Nicolette. He knew that playing in her wild, copper-tinged bush of a bohemian hairstyle was possible in the dark. He knew the scent of that jasmine body oil she wore would be just as potent without sight. No, he knew he would need to keep the lights on because of her past.

Nicolette was a dew-laden gardenia whose petals had been misused and bruised as a child from a trusted family friend. He could tell by the jarring abstract painting she entitled "Uncle" in the gallery downtown. The way she folded her arms tight to her flat chest as she stood by it. And so he bought it just to put in his storage unit and out of her sight.

Jacques sensed it all in the splashes of blue and red paint on the canvas. Now she lay naked, with her long legs of almond, on his canvas, his king-sized bed with a look of polite obligation on her face, her eyes focusing on some point in the ceiling as if in the dentist's chair.

"The painting, where is it?"

"I told you, it's in my office downtown."

Jacques set out to make a masterpiece of her, being Miles Davis during the Kind of Blue sessions, making her clit his trumpet's gleaming mouthpiece. Nicolette eventually came mid-composition in a repressed fit of thrashing about. She broke off contact with a sudden scampering back from his mouth.

"You okay?"

"Just," she draw her twitching legs together and smiled and nodded, "I'm good."

As entered her she asked him what was up with "the eyeballing," the watching her so intently. She wrinkled her nose. "Kinda creeeepy."

Jacques knew better and challenged her. "No, it isn't. You're fucking beautiful, Nicky. I want remember ever blink of her eyelash. Turn your face and close your eyes if you need to, but I'm going to take in everything about you."

Jacques began with an easy lift stroke. He curled his neck back nice and easy to emphasize the wave rolling down his spine into her. Nicolette turned her head and breathed as if meditating. He did all that he could to put as little impact onto her as possible. Focusing instead on massaging that pink gardenia.

Nicolette's breathing grew heavier. Jacques went on, yet wanted more of a response, more of a confirmation that he was more than doing her justice.

He noticed that Nicolette was rolling her hips, ever so slightly. As if she was fighting her own instincts. Yes, little signs. She exhaled out of her mouth, a little. Fingertips grazed his triceps as if determined not to full out grip them. And then again, the hips rolled. A little.

Jacques detected a hard and high roll to his left, her right hip. He closed his eyes. What could rising the right hip mean? He ran through projections of sexual geometry in his mind until he realized the raising of the hip brings more of the wall on that side in contact with his *stroke. Jacques looked down at her.*

Nicolette turned to meet his eyes. "What?"

Jacques reared back to lift her right leg up to a 90-degree angle. He sat up onto his knees, spread wide for balance, and worked lift stroke that rode her right wall. Nicolette shuddered. She turned her face to the side and inhaled deeply.

Jacques brought a light popping end to his strokes.

"Mmm," there it was, her first moan. She quickly put a hand over her mouth as if to stuff it back down her throat. Jacques moved her hand away. No.

The day trader tightened his grip of her thigh and sent a deep thrust into her right wall, letting it stick. Nicolette took a firm hold of his forearms. She looked Jacques in the eyes. He exited so slowly she sighed like someone finally coming to grips with being at the top of a rollercoaster and rush of pressure and energy that awaiting her.

Jacques placed Nicolette's leg down so that it lay across her left hip. Feeling a shift in texture of her walls from the change, he leaned back to prop himself up by his hands. Still on his knees, he braced his strokes with his hands, bringing them in on a higher curve to send her into a state long overdue.

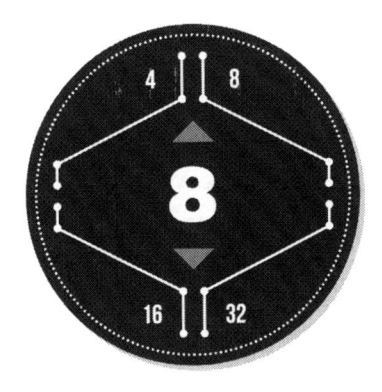

TRAINING STROKE SKILLS

There is nothing more deceptive than an obvious fact.
- Arthur Conan Doyle

In the world of fitness, there is a huge lie that the industry tells us over and over again. The lie is that strengthening specific muscles will improve form and technique applicable in other parts of your life. You have seen this and heard it before. Television ads love to show us men working out and then scoring a touchdown, shooting a ball through a hoop, or sprinting. You see it even more in articles, videos, and podcasts that advocate doing various exercises to improve your sensual skill performance.

Just Google "best exercises for sex" and you will see thousands of these articles and videos. They are misleading and can do more harm than good. A study done by Snyder, Connor, and Ebersole out of Bristol

University found that general and even targeted strength training does little to improve movement patterns associated with tasks like running or performing better in bed

…There is still a lack of consensus about how these factors would respond to different training interventions. For example, when strength training exercises were used alone, including closed-chain hip rotation, bands, machine and free weight lower body exercises, studies reported no change [5] to significant modifications [20] in the hip internal rotation, and knee abduction moment during running or cut and jump actions.[4]

In the study, they looked at glutes (butt muscles) and its crucial role in sprinting. The assumption was that by targeting and training this specific muscle, the runner would be able to run faster. They trained his glutes until they were stronger than when they started and then had him sprint the same distance. The results were that there was less than a 1% improvement.

The reason why there was so little improvement is because it was used to running a certain way. Since it is simpler to do what you are used to, you revert back to what you know best.

The sprinter was sure that he could have been faster, but he had not broken the pattern that would utilize the new strength his body had created. Let me be clear here, if you want to be good at picking up

---

4 https://www.researchgate.net/publication/23477954_Snyder_KR_Earl_JE_O'Connor_KM_Ebersole_KT_Resistance_training_is_accompanied_by_increases_in_hip_strength_and_changes_in_lower_extremity_biomechanics_during_running

weights and putting them down, then the gym is enough. However, if you plan on using your fitness for any other activity, then you need more. If you want to improve a unique ability, skill, or movement, you need to practice that movement or ability.

This was research that I did before working to develop the Tantra Bodybuilding System. It guided the construction of the entire framework of the system. Any man who wants to perform better in bed needs to practice the same motions that he would perform there. As a man wanting to improve his sensual game, you need to have a workout that:

1. Builds lean muscle

2. Builds endurance using that lean muscle

3. Builds rhythm

All these things need to occur while allowing you to train the specific movements that you would use in bed. If any of these things did not take place, then the whole program would fail. Because no one else took the time to take this research into consideration, they leave practitioners with frustrations and complications.

1. You don't ever use the strength you've built because you are training irrelevant movements.

2. You have all these things you read about but never use them because you haven't broken your old patterns.

3. You feel your muscles working against you making you look and feel more awkward and also less powerful than you did before.

Don't get me wrong; it is okay to train in exercises that develop the important movement principles that surround an activity. But when it comes to upgrading your ability to perform, nothing is going to trump actually doing that activity.

So in laymen's terms... Want better mechanics to run better? Train the mechanics to run better. Want better mechanics to trigger orgasms? Train the mechanics to trigger orgasms.

I want to give you a clear understanding of each level of this hierarchy pyramid so that you understand just how and why this type of process allows you to do the most important thing that no other fitness program or self-development program will do and that is giving you a personal relationship with your sexual physique. That means you understanding how your body works sexually and master it so that you can modify change and adapt any type of sexual situation.

This is not some type of trick or gimmick, no! This is a reintroduction to who you are. You need to know what you do well, what are your strengths and how to build on them. You need to know your weaknesses and how to turn them into strengths! Let me get right to it, because this concept of bodybuilding your sexual physique is so new that I'm going to equate everything to boxing. That way you can see the relationship between how a boxer built himself up and how you are going to build yourself up. Before you get in the ring, before you learned any punches, you build your body. Boxers move in a specific kind of way, so when you're going in and dealing with a good boxing trainer, you are prepared to do training exercises that develop the parts of your body that you're going to use the most when you're in the ring. It's the exact same thing when it comes to stroke skills.

When you start Stroke Skills, you're going to work on the parts of your body you use the most during sex. In most cases these parts of your body you have never exercised because of the fact that the whole fitness system leaves them out. That's how come you see real in shape bodybuilders they have no flexibility around their hips or the lower lumbar. They're stiff, in fact when they walk their hips don't even move, now can you imagine how terrible those guys must be in bed? No, I'm not trying to get my ass kicked, so I'm going to get off that subject and get you back to the point - which is the first step is training the parts of your body that are used most during sex.

We have a DVD called the Tantra Bodybuilding P90X for sex DVD. It's has more than 10 brand-new exercises that do nothing but build stamina and strength to the parts of your body that you use most during sex and that is your arms, your back, your lower lumbar, your psoas, your hip, your thighs and specifically your hip rotation. All of those things you have to have. We're talking about endurance, stamina so when you are making love your body won't get tired. So going back to the boxing gym analogy, after you learned to empower those different parts of your body to be a boxer you learn punches. The first punches that you learn in boxing are your jabs. The jab is used as a timekeeper used to keep your opponent at bay and is also used to measure distance which is very important because understanding distance tells you when to use a more advance punches.

In Stroke Skills, our jab are called base strokes and they have a very, very similar purpose: the base strokes give you something called perpetual or live rest. That means your body is able to move consistently inside of a woman without you becoming tired. It gives you something to do when you're inside of her so that you can actually rest while staying in motion. This is extremely important because most women lose their orgasms not because of the fact that they wouldn't get them but because of the fact that they lose stimulation and that means that we stop moving. When we stop moving they can no longer build toward the orgasm, they need constant stimulation.

Our jabs also allow you to actually launch other strokes off, just like your boxing jab allows you to launch other punches off of it. You do this consistently and when you get tired of doing your flurries with your more advance punches, you can go back to base stroking, throwing your "jab" keeping her in the game and simultaneously keeping all the energy and sexual stimulation that you created from going to waste. There is nothing more important than your base stroke. You will learn four different base strokes. In each of those base strokes give women a different type of stimulation. The idea is that all women are different and all women require a different type of base stroke. You find the one that stimulates her the way that she enjoys being stimulated. From there, you can launch other more complicated strokes that you learn later but you'll always go back to your base stroke so that you can rest.

S.T.R.O.K.E

So now, as a boxer, you have a boxer's body. Simultaneously, you have these punches that you know how to use if you were in the gym. The next thing you would learn is footwork. Footwork is what gets you in and away from your opponent. It's your footwork that keeps you from getting hit and also your footwork that puts you in the position to throw punches and actually hit back. In stroke skills your footwork is 80:10:10, your 80:10:10 is a sexual strategy that gives you different ways to manipulate depth. This strategy is going to tell you how you can use your punches to effectively build her orgasms up. You're actually creating the orgasmic experience through your 80:10:10. The way that you use your strokes for building orgasms is similar to the way that you would use your punches to create a knockout. It doesn't matter what strokes that you're using the 80:10:10 is the foundation.

So now you have a toned boxer's body, incredible jabbing punches and the footwork to get in and out of range to use those punches. What comes next? Well, if you were in a boxing gym you would learn to use those punches for different purposes. Because you can throw a punch doesn't mean that the way you're throwing the punch is going to be effective for the specific outcome that you want to have. If you throw your jab to keep your opponent at bay you're not going to throw that jab with a lot of power, no! It's going to be springy, it's going to pop and it's going to make them stay put while you move to another position however, you can also throw a jab like Tommy Hearns or Sugar Ray Leonard who have knocked people out with jabs before. That means shooting the jab with the strength and the power that actually has a knockout ability. So what we're speaking about now is inflection or the way that you manipulate something to have one effect or another.

Stroke Skills has a compression strategy and an impact strategy. They use your inflection in different ways so you can throw your strokes to evoke a different response. Women orgasm when we either use our stroke to compress a spot or to bring impact on it. A woman would have to eventually show a preference around which one she enjoys. Many women might have a different preference from day-to-day. They might like this spot compressed on one day and they might like that spot impacted one another day. The bottom line is that you know how to do both you have this strategy to be able to throw your punch in either way so that you can make sure that you bring her to that type of orgasm that she wants each and every time.

Let's take it back to the gym. We started boxing. We developed our bodies so that we can build a boxer's physique. We developed the skill to use our jab to keep timing and keep distance with our partner. We've learned to be able to maneuver around the ring so that we can follow our opponent and deliver punches exactly to the places they need to be delivered, lastly we were able to learn exactly how to deliver those punches to strike our opponent in a way that would result in a knockout. Even the most intellectual of us can recognizes the importance of this process:

It is because the body is a machine that education is possible. Education is the formation of habits, a super inducing of an artificial organization upon the natural organization of the body.

- Thomas Henry Huxley

Let us take it back to stroke skills terms. We developed our sexual physique. We've actually put time into building the muscles that are used mostly when we have sex to now these muscles are strong and flexible and they can endure, yes! Next we learned exactly how to use our muscles to stay perpetually moving when we're making love to a woman so it doesn't matter what we decide to do we can give her stimulation using our bodies and not get tired. We've learned that 80:10:10 sexual strategy so that now when we stroke we know that we are building on top of our strokes, we're not rushing. We are stroking in a way as to make her naturalized to us, it's to make her body open up to us. We know how to introduce our unique body, our unique cock to her in a way that she is going to accept and she's going to start relaxing and feeling all that friction energy building into herself.

Thanks to the 80:10:10 strategy we can get them to the point that they are full of sex energy, where their spots are full of friction energy. Since we understand now that we can either compress that spot or impact that spot due to our knowledge of how to manipulate our stroke, we can bring her to an orgasm in the type of fashion that she enjoys. Whether you're a boxer or not, you're a man that is developing his sexual physique via stroke skills. You have your foundation. All this is true, however, you couldn't call yourself a boxer and you couldn't call yourself being skilled until you do what? Train.

What would a trainer have you do in the boxing gym after you learn the basics, after you got the foundation, after you built your body to understand the base punches and how to maneuver around the ring? What would they do next? They would make you start looking in the mirror, yes! They will start making you look at yourself and check yourself out. They would say know what unique attributes you bring to the boxing arena, what do you do well. It is no different with stroke skills. After you have this foundation you could say that you know how to stroke but you wouldn't say that you were skilled until we started looking at your unique style, until we started crafting what advanced strokes, what advanced strategies and position modifications fit your body type.

You are entering an arena. Understand that it is your job as a man to leave your name and leave your sweat on the floor of that arena. You're not coming in there to be anybody else but yourself so you have to understand that you must learn yourself. That's the next and most exciting step when it comes to stroke skills. You might have large legs, you might have a bigger upper body, you might have a larger stomach, you might have a larger back. When you're building those muscles back at step one that you got with the P90 X for sex DVD you really started learning what things were best for you. Your body started moving toward certain movements and away from others. You recognized that certain things were easier for you that you enjoy more. All that comes into play later when we start saying let's capitalize on those strengths that you have.

What you focus on expands. So focus on what you want, not what you do not want.

— Esther Jno-Charles

You might have a skill where you just naturally spring in the bedroom with a natural hip-pop that you do well. Simply key in on different advance strokes that utilize that, so now when you are in the mix using your base stroke with 80:10:10 technique you're navigating her and you're bringing the stroke to her in a sequential way that has your own signature. That's right, you'll launch from your base stroke from your jab to your whole unique arsenal! You do those until your body gets a bit fatigued but you don't stop because you've trained for this. You go back to your base stroke and you can utilize that live rest - being able to stay in perpetual motion while your body rejuvenates. Always keeping the energy, keeping the sensual pleasure that you build into her going. No more letting that fall off the cliff.

You're keeping it in play so that when you finish your live rest while doing our base stroke inside of her to maintain all of that pleasure, you can launch back into your unique set, into that thing that will have you be something memorable to the utmost. She's going to remember you and she's going to know that she would never ever be able to get that type of experience anywhere else.

She could never get a replication of what you brought because what you brought was a culmination of time, muscle memory, sweat, hard work, caring, appreciation, love for yourself and dedication to making your mark as a man. It's your signature. It's yours and yours alone. At that point in time you can call yourself skilled. In fact, she is going to tell you that you are skilled, she is going to thank you for unlocking things inside of her, she's going to thank you for revealing things that she never knew about herself through the way that you have sex with her. She's going to thank you and you know what? You're going to say 'you are welcome. You did something that made me feel as though you were deserving and that was my way of appreciating you.'

I want each and every one of you to experience this. I'm a man, I'm mortal. I'm not going to have this ability to speak to you my whole life. At some point in time I'm going to go back to the dirt. I don't want to die without leaving this on the planet so that men could remember and feel what it's like to truly be a man. I want you to feel what it's like when you see them dumping Gatorade on that quarterback at the Super Bowl's end and run around the stadium. That's how it can feel that each and every night in your own home with your woman.

That's the thing that I want to have here after I'm dead and gone. I want you to be able to benefit from this work that I'm doing to bring back what true manhood feels like. We work too hard to not enjoy this. We deserve this we deserve to remember what it feels like to be a man and it all starts with you getting in touch, recognizing and learning to appreciate your own sexual physique. I want you to make your sexual physique into a hulk. I want you to be rippling with muscles, rippling with ability, poised with stamina and prepared to go whenever you want to go. When you build a foundation, everything on top of it is secure, your belief in yourself, you believe in your dreams and aspirations, your believe that you can have what you want in this life and that you deserve it.

You know that inside, stripped down naked you have something that is uniquely yours that you can give to somebody and it is potent, powerful and can never be duplicated. I want you to start this program as soon as possible make it part of your life, make this lifestyle something that you live day-to-day and you will see benefits far surpass the bedroom.

As a founder of Tantra Bodybuilding, my greatest struggle is gaining legitimacy and through it, traction with the billions of men who populate the Earth whom I know would greatly benefit from bodybuilding their sexual physique. Often when I present Tantra Bodybuilding to men, there is a bit of a pushback. The idea of improving our sexual motility is still pretty foreign as both a concept and a practice regardless of its instantaneous benefits.

Over the years, I have spoken to hundreds of bodybuilders and I figured out that I was speaking the wrong language. When I started speaking about what harm we are doing to ourselves by not having any training for our hips, they started listening up. I was able to prove that there are *no* gym exercises that activate our hips. The ones that come close can actually do more harm than good if you are not training movement along with the weight lifting.

What happens is that you can actually lose mobility/motility in your hips through weighted squats, lunges and dead lifts (the only things that come close to engaging the hips).

Men generally stiffen up and it makes them unable to perform well sexually. What's worse is that the more muscular you get, the worse it can become. Don't believe me?

Flexibility, generally speaking, is the most important physical quality. The impact of the flexibility on all other physical qualities is greater than the one of any other single physical quality. Flexibility potentially improves strength, speed and endurance more than any of these qualities impact on the other. In addition, I believe of all physical qualities, this one has the greatest impact on injury prevention. Flexibility training also potentially has the greatest contribution to recovery of all the physical qualities.[5]

Check out the strongman competition and watch how they walk. Their hips are basically non-existent. They have no mobility. I love the strongman competition, but truly feel bad for them and their girlfriends. It's sad because they're not having a diversified training regimen for their hips, which can cause these guys to get hurt and stay hurt for years (check out Louis Vondemant). The hips, hip flexors, and psoas tissue array are responsible for improvements in joint loading. Hip strengthening exercises via functional training has also been proven to reduce acute pain during exercise (specifically in the joints).

You know that joint loads are the force that your joints are under when you do activities. Joint loads contribute to wear and tear of the joint. You sometimes see a basketball player collapse to the ground in agony after leaping to grab a ball that he normally jumps and grabs with ease. You have likely seen a power lifter fold on a squat he has done a hundred times before. The issue is that their joints have overloaded without notice.

Joint loads differ according to the type of activity you engage in, your technique in doing it, and your body weight. This table shows

---

[5] http://breakingmuscle.com/mobility-recovery/flexibility-is-like-any-other-discipline-it-takes-discipline

joint loads as they relate to body weight for some common exercise activities. If, for example, you weigh 150 pounds and walk at 3 miles per hour (mph), you place 705 pounds of force on your hip joint (4.7 multiplied by 150) with every step. If you run at 7 mph, the load is 900 pounds.

As you can see, weightlifters are at extreme risk for having joint failure even with supplementation for joint lubrication. Hip strengthening is one of the only activities that lead to improvements in joint loading.

In a study headed by Dr. Kimberly L. Dolak, MS, ATC[1]:

Subjects who started with hip strengthening reported an earlier and more significant drop in knee pain after only 4 weeks of rehabilitation, while the patients who initially performed quadriceps strengthening required 8 weeks of rehabilitation to achieve a similar decrease in pain.

Your current exercise isn't going to cut it for you. Researchers agree that those who are active in running, weight training, skiing, or other physical activities have a lot of inherent movement intelligence that make it harder to improve.

The body adapts to move in the path of least resistance *(not necessarily the best or safest path – just the easiest)* and when something might change this preferred movement pattern *(like changes in joint forces from stronger muscles),* the body simply adapts to maintain its old pattern and can become even more challenging to correct as you age. As we get older we actually end up with less and less range of motion because we do less and less. Think about it - if you're twenty years old, you'll have spent about fourteen years sitting down (enter school at age six and then spend most of your time at a desk during school hours and then again for homework, plus add in time spent sitting for meals, travel, and activities like video games). But, if you're forty, you'll have accumulated 34 years of spending a majority of your time sitting. All that time spent sitting tells your body that it only needs to work in a limited range, that the hips only ever need to be at roughly at ninety degrees, that it's normal for the upper body to hunch and the shoulders to round. Just like if you spent 34 years punching a bag and your body got really good at punching the bag, you're spending lots and lots of time on reps that make your body really good at being in the seated position.[6]

---

6   Ibid

You need something new. A series of functional training activities prior to exercising will allow you to lift more, lift healthier, and lift more confidently so that your gym regimen won't result in you needing to use a cane.

You could look at the bedroom benefits as a bonus. At least until you use them. At which point, you will likely see the assistance it gives to your gym regimen and joint maintenance as your second and third favorite features.

> **Phil** → Grace · 2 years ago
> OMG! I laughed when I read this. But it is SO TRUE! I'm getting married April 20th 2013. And my girl told the me exact same thing. That I need to learn how to gyrate my hips in bed. I said WHAT!? So did what any other computer nerd does, I researched the life out of it. And I found Zenity Fitness. There's many sexual fitness exercises to this.
>
> And WOW! Am I learning. I've lost 30 pounds and my hips are strong and loose.
>
> How I know it's working, because my lady stares at me doing my plank position hip exercises, it involves "rhythm hip movements". It's like sensual hypnosis as she watches, and she loves it.
> ∧ | ∨ · Reply · Share ›

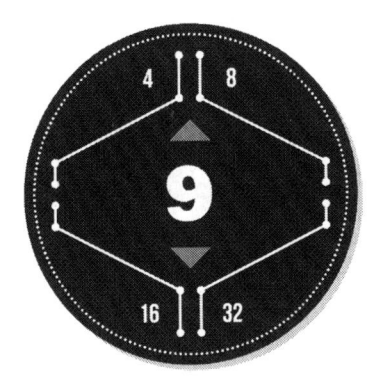

RHYTHM MOVEMENT & THE OCEAN

Communication leads to community, that is, to understanding, intimacy and mutual valuing. - Rollo May

All the clichés about the "motion of the ocean" are true when it comes to sex positions. Regardless of what sex position you're in, regardless of how big your penis might be, if there's no rhythm or if you and your partner can't get in synch, the penetration is going to destroy the moisture and along with it the opportunity for orgasm. This makes the ability to synch your rhythm to your partner's an invaluable skill that should be developed and honed on your own time.

Why? Because sex isn't the practice for the big game. It *is* the big game. You train for sex so that you can perform at your A level. It is not the time to be thinking, it's time to be doing.

This means your rhythm development is something you want to invest in and perfect. Learning to move to a rhythm can very well be one of the most awkward experiences of a lifetime for many people. However, I have taught many guys to do it, and many of them had two left feet (or two left hips in this case). Even though people say that you either have rhythm or you don't, in reality, we all have rhythm. Some of us just require more focus to realize it.

rhythm
(noun)
1. a strong, regular, repeated pattern of movement or sound.

synonyms: pattern, flow, tempo

"the rhythm of daily life"

2. the systematic arrangement of musical sounds, principally according to duration and periodic stress.

synonyms: beat, cadence, tempo, time, pulse, throb, swing

"the rhythm of the music"

3. a particular type of pattern formed by rhythm.

"guitar melodies with deep African rhythms"

Rhythm is actually engrained in your nervous system and since your nervous system also plays a huge part in when we have sex, the two are naturally intertwined. Think about the last time you kept a pace or a beat when intimate. In whatever position you were in, you delivered thrusts in a sequence that likely went 1-2-3-4. When you did this, your nervous system kicked in and let you feel the pleasure associated with your thrusts. Now, what if I told you her nervous system did the same thing... It is true, since we are inside of a woman, she also feels and associates pleasure with rhythm. It's why women will say that they like it fast or slow. They associate those paces with a pleasurable sensation.

Now imagine you could build variations on slow and fast to key into exactly the kind of sensations that are uniquely pleasurable to her vagina (exciting right? We will get to that).

You have rhythm and you have used it... Now how can we turn it up?

The answer is in the spinal cord, specifically in your hips, which have a direct connection to your psoas and actionable ligaments in your pelvis. These networks are called Central Pattern Generators, or CPGs.

Basically, CPGs coordinate your muscles so that they work in a perfect sequence to make walking very easy and efficient. Therefore, all you have to do is think: "walk." Of course, it's never this black and white; our brains regulate our walking substantially and we react to our senses to make adjustments (like stepping on a rock). Nevertheless, the basic pattern comes from activating these little networks.

So what does this have to do with your Stroke Skills?

It turns out that these CPGs can be adapted and utilized for different rhythms and patterns.

To quote the author in the reference above: *"As animals mature, there are changes in the rhythmic motor patterns they express. For instance, tadpoles swim, but frogs hop; chicks hatch, but then walk; humans crawl, then walk, then run. Furthermore, humans can easily learn novel rhythmic motor patterns (e.g. swimming strokes, dances) that, once learned, seem as 'automatic' and ingrained as do clearly CPG-driven motor patterns such as walking."*

Those of us who train in Tantra Bodybuilding already know that when it comes to practicing strokes, once you get the rhythm, your muscle memory locks on and then you can do it almost automatically without thinking of the details.

You can literally just think the name and your hips will do it and your mind will be aware of it. This is an experience that we all can have because we all have these CPG networks in our nervous systems. Therefore, it just takes practice, and you *will* learn to stroke on rhythm.

We have created a unique kind of assistance for helping you to practice, which makes it impossible to not be on beat. It is called a Stroke Tracking Rhythm.

Use Stroke Tracking Rhythms to perfectly time out your stroke routine, allowing you to choose a rhythm to stroke to within the 4 minutes of song play. Each track gives you 10 seconds of prep time to set up and choose your rhythmic/auditory goal.

1. Tracking: Track her rhythm

2. Flowing: Change the rhythm when she does

3. Pinning: Intuitively attach a specific stroke when her body asks for it.

From there, you simply follow the instrumental music and focus in on your intent; whether you are **Tracking, Flowing, or Pinning**. It works because you instantly recognize that you are doing it and then you will start to key into micro rhythms.

You will start realizing what rhythm you are naturally drawn to and then how to switch on and off of the rhythm (because sometimes you don't want to be predictable with your stroke). Feels awkward? Of course it does. But feeling awkward is a good thing. Besides, it's much better to feel awkward while practicing than while performing.

Just keep stroking and eventually it will feel as natural as walking.

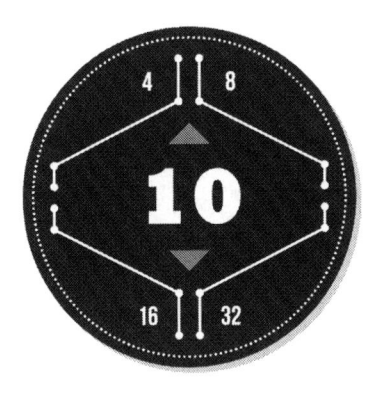

RHYTHM TRAINING

Life is about rhythm. We vibrate, our hearts are pumping blood, we are a rhythm machine, that's what we are. - Mickey Hart

One thing that makes Zenity very unique is the fact that rhythm plays a key role in our fitness concept. It is this way for two specific reasons. The first reason deals with the fact that the body makes processes easier the more that you do them. Even when we build this sexual muscle memory, we want the body to be able to perform these stroking exercises with far less strain and far less trouble. With each of these movements, we want them to be able to perform them with ease. However, when it comes to the fitness element, we want their muscles to continue to grow. That means that we have to change the rhythm occasionally so that the body cannot rely on that muscle memory to make it easier.

People tend to play in their comfort zone, so the best things are achieved in a state of surprise, actually. - Brian Eno

We want it to be easy in the bedroom, we don't necessarily want it to be easy in the gym because they won't grow. They will not see the definition. They will not see the strength increases that they want if their body allows them to cheat. Your body is intelligent; it wants you to work less and spend less energy and it is going to do what it can to achieve that. To offset this, we deal with rhythm differentiation simply because when we do this it changes the way that the muscles have to work in order to do the exercise. That means that even though the muscle memory is still there, you are still having to perform some extra exertion in order to do these exercises. This allows us to give people the physical results that they want.

I said there were two reasons. The second reason is that it's imperative that we understand how to perform our strokes on a rhythm - specifically on the rhythm that our partner is interested in. Women close to an orgasm will require a man to stroke to a certain depth at a certain location in their body, however they have to continue that stroke at a certain pace or the woman will completely lose their orgasm. It is no different vice versa; if a woman is stroking a man, it's the consistency of her stroke that allows him to go further into the feeling and then climax from that consistency. Being able to maintain a rhythm and being able to pick up a rhythm and hold the pace are the finer points of what makes someone good in bed.

Now nobody in the world deals with this except us at Zenity, so this information that you are receiving now is extremely rare and equally powerful. What is even more potent is the way that we train those abilities into people. A lot of people naturally have rhythm, but many people don not; you treat both the same. We have three different elements that we use to train rhythm at Zenity. I am going to go through each element and briefly explain why that element is so important.

The first rhythm training element is called tracking. Tracking is important because it teaches a man or a woman how to sync with their partner. With tracking you want to play music with a very basic and consistent beat; you want to start with something slower when your client first engages you but then as you move forward from week to week, you play music that has a faster pace. But you want the beat to be consistent and relatively easy to pick up on. You want to have your client to stroke to that beat. They are performing their exercises to that beat.

You can demonstrate for them so that they see how to perform whatever exercises you are dealing with to that rhythm because it's going to teach them about rhythm and about the whole idea of syncing your stroke to a specific and unique rhythm. Is that clear? Good. The purpose for this sexually is to get your partner to understand how to ride a rhythm when their partner demonstrates it. In many cases what happens is that when you're having sex with somebody, your partner will basically submit a certain rhythm that they enjoy; they will actually start moving at a rhythm they appreciate. With this type of training you teach yourself how to sync to your partner's rhythm and stay with it.

In many cases the thing that is going to happen in a sexual situation is when you are able to sync with your partner's rhythm, at some point in time they are going to change it, meaning at some point in time their rhythm will change. So what we do is have another rhythm training concept that allows people to understand how to change rhythms. You don't want to pigeonhole someone into one ability; you want to give them the flexibility to move and meander between different skills or tempos. We train these men and women on how to switch rhythms while they are stroking and to do this, we have a type of training called Flow Training.

Flow Training is unique because it uses a specific type of music that was created at Zenity fitness. This music has a multitude of different kinds of beats playing simultaneously. It will have drums playing simultaneously with different rhythm patterns with different guitar riffs. You play this music and allow your client to perform the stroke that you are discussing. When you give the signal, you tell them to switch rhythm and they would go from stroking to one beat that's inside of this music to the other. They might have been stroking to a bass drum and then you would say "okay, now stroke to the guitar," and now they change their pace. They have to change their rhythm and modify the stroke accordingly. It could be faster or slower. This creates a skill in your client so when he is intimate with his partner and his muscle memory is locking into her rhythm. Should she change, the muscle memory changes with her. It is going to be subconscious; he or she won't even have to think about it. Her body will do it, leaving them to focus on their partner and the experience.

The third section of the audio training that Zenity features is called pinning. Pinning is all about training personal inflection, and what does that mean you ask? Personal inflection, when it comes to your Zenity training, would be how you choose to employ which of the skills that you have developed to use? You have several and they are all in your muscle memory; they are all locked into your memory banks. What impetus or type of motivation do you need to be able to choose one versus the easiest one? This is demonstrated easily in martial arts where people not trained to actually use the various arsenals of martial arts skills that they have, when in a real confrontation, use the one that they use the most and a lot of times is going to be the most basic.

So, you have all these different skills as martial artist, as a fighter and you get into a real combat situation and the only thing that you can remember to do is to punch, regular old punch; but you are a black belt. That would be a defeatist type of modality if we had that same type of mind-set when it comes to Zenity.

The whole Zenity format is features exercises that are functional in bed. We want men and women to use them in bed, and so we have to teach them how to use them. By teaching them how, we have to find a way to evoke their use of more than one of the skills. They have to have a reason to dig deeper and truly show the different things that they have. Now our solution for this is pinning.

In pinning you would use music that has very sporadic type of beats; it's not consistent, it doesn't use any type of regular consistent rhythm; no, this is sound effects, there are horns, there are trumpets that are coming out of various different places. You can't expect what is going to happen. And you tell your client to move based on what they feel; listen to the sound and do a movement from an arsenal that represented that sound. You tell them to move with it; you tell them to try to pin a movement; pin a stroke to the sound; turn up the music and let them go.

So what you have done in this point in time is that you have ensured that your training is going to be effective. You have ensured that they will see results. You have programmed them to believe in themselves.

Now in the package that you received with your instructor training, you are going to get a guide that's going to break it all down. I wanted to speak about in audio because your understanding is what's most important and sometimes I think that when somebody speaks, you can hear their passion and really get focused as opposed to simply reading something. Sure, you can go and check out the manual. I have more bulleted type of information there when it comes to these three sections. But the rhythmic concept within Zenity of tracking; being able to track her rhythm; flow, being able to change the tempo and style of their rhythm when they change it and pinning, being able to train yourself to develop your own rhythm and furthermore use the arsenal of skills that you have had. These different elements you can weave into your practice, into your sessions with your client to make things more fun, to shake things up, so to speak.

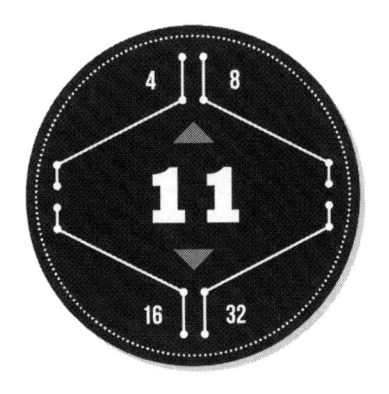

SEXUAL GEOMETRY

I think the universe is pure geometry - basically, a beautiful shape twisting around and dancing over space-time. - Antony Garrett Lisi

The people that brought positions to us are not as good as we are in bed. They were terrible then. They were absolutely terrible. In this day and age, we are the best sexually that we've ever been. As men, and we have to remember that in order to be able to become and reach the potential that we have, we have to go back and rip out the floorboards that are rotting the foundation of our sexual understanding. What does that analogy mean? It means that we have things that have been embedded into us that keep us from being able to truly recognize our potential and in order to recognize that potential we have to go back and we have to remove that information that is keeping us from our greatness. Comprehending the importance of sexual movement is one of the things that we have to do in order to reach our potential.

Additionally, we actually have an interest in pleasing women, when in the past men really didn't even have a reason to please women. It was all about the conquest of them and operating on them versus with them for their pleasure. In the past it's been about operating **on** them versus **with** them. But today we have enough information to change all that, and as I said understanding sexual movement as being a foundation of everything sexual as it pertains to intercourse is something that we need to truly focus on.

This segment is going to take you through five different steps in understanding the concept of sexual geometry. It's going to move through quickly because the idea is for you to get this information and put it to use and not be spending all your time listening to me.

The first area is going to be called: *Your penis as a massage tool*. In this area you're going to hear about the dimensions and concepts of using your penis as a way of massaging a woman from the inside. It's going to completely change the ideas around positions. Please understand the full concept of what I mean when I say massage.

massage

noun

1.

the rubbing and kneading of muscles and joints of the body with the hands, especially to relieve tension or pain.

"massage can ease tiredness and jet lag"

verb

1.
rub and knead (a person or part of the body) with the hands.
"he massaged her tired muscles"

2.
manipulate (figures) to give a more acceptable result.
"the accounts had been massaged and adjusted to suit the government"

Second, *how to use the guide*. You have a comprehensive guide that's coming and this section is going to tell you about how to use that guide effectively to benefit your relationship and how to put it to use immediately.

Third, *Missionary is your starting point*. This area is going to speak about the missionary position and how you can master missionary and use it to be able to master all the other positions.

Lastly, *Building a foundation*. This area is going to tell you exactly how you can start to acquire a multitude of different skills, just as a boxer acquires a multitude of different punches. The idea being that you learn these punches and discover how they specifically work with your body so that you learn to throw them and use them in a unique way, except these punches that we'll be teaching are actually sexual movement processes called strokes that will change the way that your lady feels about you forever. I'm truly excited about sharing this information with you. I can guarantee that this is the only place in the world that you will read about sexual geometry and the importance of sexual movement. On to the first area, *Your penis as a massage tool*.

The word penis sounds so technical. I like to use the penis simply because it sounds a lot more masculine and debonair, and our penis is both masculine and debonair. Bear with me as I use this term through the duration of this course.

First and foremost, how do you define your penis? Do you look at it as an organ or do you look at it as a massage tool? Now most of you will not look at it as a massage tool because of the fact we don't look at our bodies and our way that we interact with women as a pleasure device. When we become sexual with the woman our body literally becomes the most intricate, high-tech vibrator that the world will ever know. Yes, the rabbit, the dolphin, the bullet, none of these vibrators will never be able to touch us. Why? Because we are thinking, intelligent and interactive vibrators, and our penis is an expandable cylinder that can be used not just to target spots in a women's body but to actually help her find spots that she never knew existed.

There are two ways that you find spots in a woman's body. One way is through impact and the other is through compression. I'm going to speak about impact and compression more when we talk about *Building a foundation*. Right now, I'm going to discuss exactly how you as a man should start thinking about your penis and start thinking about the action that your penis plays when it comes to sex. It will ultimately change the way that you engage women and will perpetually keep you improving as you get older. A woman's vagina has four different walls. It has four different walls and each of these walls hold various different sensitivities based upon that specific woman. Women feel pleasure because we are able to create friction by moving our penis inside of her in different ways so that the walls that are the sensitive walls are able to absorb that friction through the concept of heat. Through that heat they experience pleasure.

If you want to get a small idea of what this feels like, take your thumb and drive it into your forearm. Push down hard as you can and then skate your thumb forward towards your hand. Do you feel that hot sensation? That is exactly what we generate inside a woman when we move our penis. The key in pleasuring a woman is in finding the wall and the right pressure in which to apply that friction and heat. We do that through a process that we call the 80-10-10/spot locator technique, and this is something else that I'll speak about when we go over Building a Foundation. Right now, just try to frame that idea that she has these four walls and your penis is a massage tool that you are using to massage these four walls.

Earlier I spoke about understanding that some walls are more sensitive than others. This is why we need different ways to massage walls where one wall will get more pressure than another. Often, when a woman wants to stop having sex it's because either a wall is getting too much stimulation or not enough. A woman's body has 100 times the ability to sense pleasure than a man's does, so trust and believe that if you are doing it right she's going to want to experience that. In fact, she's going to relax and let you take control.

Now what you do when you have that control is truly the master stroke when it comes to sex, because you have the ability to stimulate different types of orgasms through various strokes - systematically tactile rhythmically organized kinetic exercises. In layman's terms, they're thrusting patterns that apply different amounts of pressure and different depths and different patterns rhythmically. They stimulate different orgasms, vaginal orgasms, clitoral orgasms, A-spot orgasms, outer vaginal orgasms and combination orgasms that can result in multiple orgasms. Again, we'll go through all this when we talk about the Foundation. Just visualize the power that you have right here and right now.

You just have to unlock the ability. It's inside of you, in fact you do a lot of it just through intuition, through feeling this woman out. You do it best with the unique body that you have. So the penis that you have, the penis that you have, you're going to be the best with it because that's the one that you've had for the most time. You've had the most experience with it. You know it better than you would if you had a different one. So the idea is that you master the ability to use it at a high, high level and you consistently upgrade. You consistently take yourself back to the boxing gym and add new punches and combinations onto your arsenal so they never know what to expect. In moments of brilliance, you can catch yourself doing moves like Jordan, making ways to score out of seemingly impossible situations. Your so-called opponent may find herself taunting you with the tearful prayer that you indeed conquer the moment.

Your penis as a massage tool. Every woman has a specific code opens everything to you if you choose the proper sequence. Unbridled gratitude and praise await when you do so.

> **Bill Green** Ha ha ha! man it is always about skills + emotions. I did some moves on a chick that I was really feeling and she lost her mind!! I loved it though because I had already lost mine before we ever kssed!! LOL!!!!
> Just now · Like

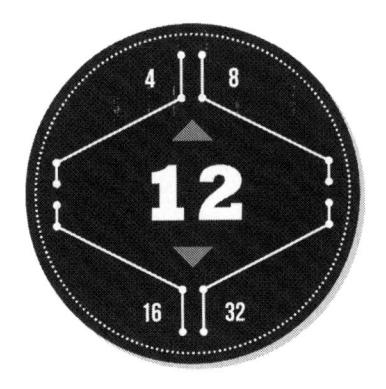

POSITIONS ARE AUTOMATIC ANGLES

All our knowledge begins with the senses, proceeds then to the understanding, and ends with reason. There is nothing higher than reason. - Immanuel Kant

An angle is essentially a place or direction that your penis is pointing based upon a way that you are positioned on a woman. Based upon the way that you are actually engaged inside of a woman and the way that her body is placed and the way that your body is placed, your penis is going to point or lean in one direction or another. It can point up, it can point down, it can point left, and it can point right. It gives you a starting point on an angle. It automatically applies a certain amount of pressure to one wall and minimize pressure to another wall. That is truly what a position is when it comes to sexual intercourse.

angle

Noun

- the space (usually measured in degrees) between two intersecting lines or surfaces at or close to the point where they meet.

- a particular way of approaching or considering an issue or problem.

There are three specific reasons why it is imperative for you to understand the concept of angles. First, all of our bodies would actually be best at certain angles versus other angles because of our height, because of our thickness, size and strength, we're going to actually feel good at certain angles versus others. We need to pay attention to our bodies and get a sense of where we are most effective. We have to lock into that mobility that angle and position is one that we can actually work from.

If you have a position where you do not feel that your body is capable of moving efficiently, then that position is not one that you should use. Simple as that. Truth be told, the position is not as important as the movement and the friction you're creating.

This leads us into the second point, which is that it's truly important that for whatever position that you decide to use, you recognize what angle in which you are pointing. Up is down, left is right and right is left. Is that clear? If you turn to the left, your cock is going to point to the right. If you turn to the right, your cock is going to point to the left. If you push your hips forward and up towards the ceiling your cock is going to point straight down, and it you point your hips down towards the ground, your cock is going to point straight up. This shows you that it doesn't matter which position that you're in, you'll know exactly which wall your penis is engaging.

This brings us to number three, and this is the thing that I truly need you to grasp. Listen to this part as many times as needed for comprehension. It'll change everything if you can get it. There's no reason to use any special positions unless you know that you're using a position that is going to be engaging a wall that you already know is pleasurable to her. Let me say that again. There's no reason to use any position unless you know that using that position will allow you to engage a wall that she already has expressed pleasure in. In other words, stick with what works.

The missionary position is your start because from missionary position you're going to do three different things:

1. You're going to find out the style of love making that she likes. Does she like a more slow style? Does she like a more pressure driven style? Does she like a more aggressive style? Does she like a more intimate style? This is going to tell you exactly the way that you want to use your body to make her feel regardless of position.

2. It's going to tell you which walls are pleasurable because from the missionary position you can effectively add pressure to every single wall. It's the only position you can do this from. You can add pressure to every single wall that exists from the missionary position. So you'll know that when you want to

transfer into other positions, you'll chose positions that will make your penis engage walls that she's already expressed a pleasure interest in. You need to master the missionary position. Mastering the missionary position opens up the reasons to use other positions.

3. STROKE. STROKE stands for Systematically Tactile Rhythmically Organized Kinetic Exercises. Strokes are the way that you move in and out of a woman. They're the different patterns, they're the different pressure systems. When I said that you can create the same sensations that any positions create from the missionary, I was speaking about using strokes from the missionary position. Strokes give you patterns that massage specific walls in specific ways and give women specific sensations. These strokes make you feel different to her. Earlier we talked about your penis, your penis being an expandable cylinder, a cylinder that expands at 360 degrees, thanks to different strokes.

Now until recently, because of books like The Kama Sutra and other books of that nature, people thought that your penis could only feel one way or another. That's because there was no concept of stroking. Now that we have the technology, we know that we can make our penis feel various different ways. We can make it feel larger, we can make it feel more compact, we can make it feel rougher, and we can make it feel smoother. We can use it to target different areas, different spots.

When you have an arsenal of strokes, when you have all these extra skills in your arsenal and you start out in that missionary position, it gives you the ability to do the research that will tell you exactly what type of feeling she will desire from you. You can then figure out what type of friction pattern feels good on which wall by cycling through your strokes and paying attention to her response. She's going to tell you with her body which one that she likes or which two that she likes.

Let's say you've had an encounter with a specific woman, starting off with the missionary in order to get your bearings. For some reason the next time you two hook up, you're feeling adventurous and you want to use a different position outside of the missionary position. Guess what? When you do that you already know what positions to choose because you know which walls she likes to be pressured. You already know which style of stroke to use because you figured that out when you were in the missionary position. So when you change to a different position you're just carrying that stroke over. You're going to be dealing with the exact same wall, you're going to be dealing with the exact same rhythm, and you're going to be going at it with the exact same intent.

It pays to have an arsenal of skills, an arsenal replete with strokes first and foremost. Then comes positions, strategies, and methodologies of connectivity. Creating a signature style evolves from this. These are all different aspects you can mix and match to keep your situation with the woman fresh. These allow you to track a woman as she changes because a woman's body will change. It will change. It's inevitable. It's only a problem if you don't have the tools to track the change and can keep that pleasure with her consistent. You want to add as many strokes into your arsenal as possible. They lock into your muscle memory and you can use them whenever needed.

Over time, you want to add as many strategies, impact strategies, compression strategies, G-spot strategies, clitoral strategies. You want to add all these things into your arsenal because they're just different ways that you can use your strokes to trigger different types of orgasms. This is what makes us as men unique. We can make love to women intelligently, using things like positions, strategies and strokes, purposefully, deliberately. It's all about mastering our bodies as the ultimate vibrator, the extreme sexual AI, picking things up about her body and how to do things to her and how to make her feel different sensations she would never ever be able to communicate to us through words.

Sex is not something where you 'just do it'. It has several significant functions associated with it. Though primarily it is meant for pleasure and satisfaction, it is just as much a physical process as a mental, emotional and psychological one. Physical involvement alone is not enough for a perfect sexual act. It demands mental, emotional and psychological involvement as well. Just as good sex generates so many happy feelings in partners, bad sex results in negative and depressing feelings. Good sex stimulates active blood circulation, burns calories and activates every part of the body, and, of course, brings the partners closer and relaxes them. Bad sex exhausts the partners to a fruitless ending and leads to frustration and emptiness in the end.

About 75 percent of all women never reach orgasm from intercourse alone -- that is without the extra help of sex toys, hands or tongue.

And 10 to 15 percent never climax under any circumstances. The Internet is rife with non-orgasmic women who say they are missing out, and statistics suggest that they are a significant group. "Maybe my boyfriend and I aren't doing it right or something," one woman wrote on WebMD.com. "I don't understand. I feel like less of a woman because I can't have an orgasm and I want to so bad. I feel incomplete sometimes after sex."[7]

If so many good feelings are associated with good sex, why not practice it in its perfect and excellent form? It's not easy to perform a perfect sexual act. It demands proper knowledge of various aspects of the sexual act. However, nothing is impossible if you have interest and desire to master it as an art.

The basics of the process are simple but the nuances make it a craft to be mastered. Above all, it's about an ability to listen to your body and watch your partner's reaction carefully.

According to sexologists (which ones?), the sexual adaptation, on average, takes six months. It must be borne in mind that the primary role for women in relationships is played by their psychological component. If a woman is psychologically content with a relationship, she will give everything to treasure that relationship. On the other hand, if she is psychologically not content with a relationship, she is unable to do so. So, to start with, you must fulfill your woman's psychological needs, otherwise you can't take your relationship forward. Simply said, if there is dissatisfaction with a partner, it can affect the quality of sex.

---

[7] http://abcnews.go.com/Health/ReproductiveHealth/sex-study-female-orgasm-eludes-majority-women/story?id=8485289

Point blank, handle your business on all fronts. Being the man in bed will not excuse neglected areas indefinitely. As far as sex is concerned, I have included some terms to facilitate a better understanding of some of the nuances this new understanding of our role requires.

Sherlocking

What is Sherlocking?

Sherlocking is the process of investigating erogenous zones and gauging stimuli that is pleasurable to your partner. The data collected by Sherlocking builds the foundation for a knowledge base.

What are Erogenous Zones?

erogenous

adjective

1. producing sexual excitement or libidinal gratification when stimulated : sexually sensitive

2. of, relating to, or arousing sexual feelings

You can find erogenous zones all over, but they tend to be located where the skin is the most sensitive. That makes sense since skin is our largest sensory organ.

Erogenous zones can often be found placed where skin is the most sensitive: the mouth, the earlobe, the nipples, the underarms, the inner surface of the shoulders and forearms, on the outer genitals, the backbone region, on the neck, around the navel, where the pubic hair begins, in the entire genital region, on the inner surface of the hips, in the crook of the elbows, behind the knees, on the feet, between the fingers and toes.

Erogenous zones are placed where skin verges on mucous membrane: lips reddening contours, nostrils' edges, vulvar lips, anal region, surface of the vulva (vagina).

Pleasure depends not as much on the stimulation technique as on our desire to have sex and our passion for our partner. There is no direct connection between caressing and excitement. Stimulation of an erogenous zone sends an impulse to the brain and only then to the hypophysis - the main sexual gland. If a woman does not want to have sex with her partner, her mind can block the tactile impulses, not allowing them to reach the hypophysis, resulting in the so-called "turning-off" of an erogenous zone and vice- versa.

Erogenous zones form a kind of map of the body, a map that should be carefully studied by the partner. One woman may have super-sensitive breasts, another may hardly react to a touch there. One woman likes to be caressed for a long time, beginning with her head and then all the way down to her feet before she is ready for sex; another just needs her fingers to be kissed. Stroke them and your partner's reaction will tell you which of them are the most sensitive. If there was no result from stimulating this or that zone, "work" with the others and you will definitely find out those delicate, responsive places that should be caressed.

To achieve the best results in the art of Sherlocking, the partner canvases the most sensitive zones and, each time, uses different kinds of caresses to determine their sensitivity. This is possible only if you are patient and sensitive to your partner. Skilled sherlocking is a real strength!

Preparation/ Platforming

First-class lovers can use their Sherlocking skills to find their partner's erogenous zones without a compass and a map and skillfully make use of these supersensitive areas to give and receive pleasure. However, as stated before, no two women are alike. Now getting them in the mood or frequency to allow you to do some Sherlocking is a preparation necessary for you both to understand each other at a level that will take the relationship to new heights. In a healthy relationship, each party should make a concentrated effort to satisfy the needs (mental, emotional, and physical) of the other person. If some of your needs aren't met, you should:

1. Examine whether you're adequately meeting the needs of the other person, and if not, make the needed adjustments.

2. Establish whether or not the needs of each person are basically compatible.

3. Decide whether a satisfying compromise can be reached.

If all of these are attempted and nothing works, then the couple may need professional help or simply incompatible through no fault of their own.

Take some initiative and do a few extra things that she normally gets done: chores, errands and so on, just to give her a bit more time for herself. It may make you look more compassionate and considerate in her eyes, and could alleviate other pressures that may be subconsciously impacting her sex drive. Don't do it expecting anything, though. Do it because it will make her feel good. Any benefit you get beyond that, should be looked upon as the cherry on top of the whipped cream.

Also attempt to make out for 5-10 minutes every day or so. No expectations. If something more happens, great, but don't be pushy. Just enjoy it together. This will really help build or repair intimacy

The 30-Day Sex Challenge, which is exactly what it sounds like. You agree to have sex for 30 days in a row, in an effort to jumpstart both the intimacy level and libido. Most women need foreplay and cuddle time afterwards. Discuss being more sexual in some place that is relaxing and non-pressured, like in the bathtub with candles.

Understand her period. Keep a diary for your own reference of when PMS starts, when she has her period (pay attention to trash cans), and note that what works sensually at this time. During this time of the month, what worked on your woman at 3:00 probably won't work at 10:00. However, it might work at 3:00 regularly…Sherlock it! Being able to help stimulate pleasure during a time when she is devoid of it, has to look really good to her and it likely makes you look very special, to say the least.

SHERLOCKING

Warming them up

It starts with the voice. Verbal stroking is the primer that should paint the walls of a room before anything goes in it. Verbal stroking aims at making your partner comfortable with the areas of their bodies they might feel uneasy about. To do this, you can just assure them that you like the way it feels, tastes, smells, looks and so on. Be sincere and watch them relax. There is a verbal stroking course offered by Stroke Skills that can elaborate on more advanced effective verbal stroking. Without putting their bodies at ease, stimulation after Sherlocking won't give them any pleasure. It will only make the process more disconcerting.

Waking Them Up

Yes, the element of surprise and variety can garner exciting results. For instance, stroke the areas surrounding the zone. Blow a thin stream of cool air across it, then breathe warm air on it. Massage the back slightly and scratch it lightly with your nails at the same time. Often, rough and intense caressing suppresses, but does not increase a woman's sensitivity. However, there are exceptions: in this case, try light pinching/slapping, let her tell you what you need to know from there.

Engaging them

Erogenous zones can be stimulated with more than hands. To increase the effect, caress them with your lips, tongue, nose and teeth. Your

S.T.R.O.K.E

partner may like you to graze her sides and inner thighs lightly. If so, experiment with a silk scarf: running it over the perineum you will excite your partner rather delicately and effectively. A vibrator can be used for the stimulation of erogenous zones if you are comfortable.

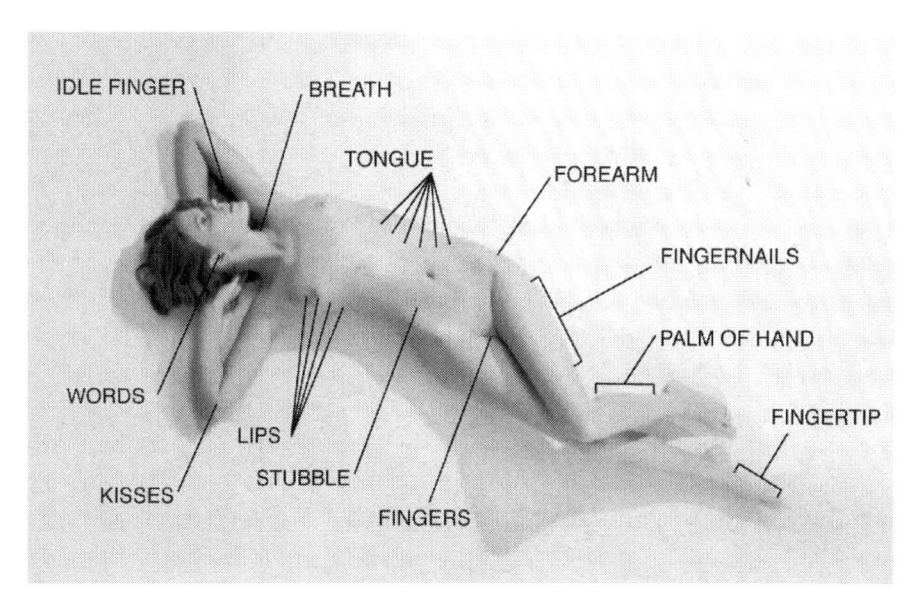

Hair and Scalp

You can run your fingers through a girl's hair. This is a great way of releasing the endorphins and is brilliant to do when you are kissing her on the lips. She will be raring to go even before you have explored the rest of her body.

Ears

Don't forget that ears are a great area to be stimulated. You have a few options here - nibble, lick or bite - but ignore them at your peril. There are lots of nerve endings in and around the ear lobe and it's a very quick way of getting your lover turned on. Be sure to give this area your attention and why not arouse this area while stimulating the head and touching her hair at the same time.

Lips

Any good lover knows that women love to be kissed and there is no getting away from it. You can keep her on her toes by incorporating different techniques. Why not try biting her bottom lip softly or pulling away at the last minute and teasing her? Have fun trying out different things and mixing it up.

Neck

This is a great area to shower her with kisses! Pay particular attention to the area 3 inches down from the earlobe and you can even kiss the jaw line. Why not try and blow your hot breath on her neck? This will make her heart miss a beat and really start turning her on.

Hands and Arms

If you want to show off your skills and let her know who she is dealing with, then don't forget the hands and arms. Ok, so it's not the most sensitive of erogenous zones but she will enjoy it and it's well worth paying attention to the little details of your lover's body. Try sucking her fingers and pay particular attention to the inside of the elbows.

Back

This is a great way to please your lover. Why not get her to lie on her stomach as you kiss and caress every part of her back? Try running your tongue down the entire length of her back, to really give her chills. Like any classic, the massage never goes out of fashion and is a great starting place when it comes to pleasing any women. Get some books and read up on the subject and don't forget the massage oils. Consider the Kama Sutra Massage Oil Serenity.

Buttocks

Approach this one with an open mind. Stimulating your lover's buttocks can be anything from a light kiss, a grab with your hands or even a good spanking session. If she likes to be spanked, then we recommend the Large Leather Paddle as its great at stimulating the erogenous zones in the buttocks. Either way she will probably love some sort of attention down there, and it is easy for transition from stimulating the back to the ass.

Stomach

The stomach can be a tricky one if she is ticklish but, usually, the more aroused you are, the less ticklish you become. It's well worth your time to explore this area in intimate detail. Why not try kissing and licking her stomach? It's a great way of teasing her as you can slowly work your way down her body. For that added heightened sensation, why not try a Pom Pom Feather Tickler made from real marabu feathers? This is an incredible experience that she will never forget and much more delicate than your fingers could ever be.

Legs

Don't forget about the legs! They are such an underrated area of a woman's body and most guys dive straight to the honey pot. Valuable time spent here will be rewarded later. Kiss, stroke and touch the insides of her thighs as this will really get her stimulated.

Feet

You either love them or hate them, but whichever way you look at it, you have an erogenous zone down there. This is quite a controversial area of the body and might best be saved for special occasion. It's great when you have just stepped out of the shower. Why not try using the Pom Pom Feather Tickler on this area and see her reaching that heavenly place?

Breasts

Did you know that a woman can experience orgasms just through having her breasts stimulated? This is because the nipples share the same "party line" that connects to the vagina. Try and mix things up a bit and don't just focus entirely on the nipples as the sides of the breasts have sensations as well. Lick, bite and kiss are all good things to do here.

Genitals

Ok, this is the number one spot for turning on your lover. Spending quality time on all the other areas to drive your partner wild are merely the opening acts before the concert's headliner. There are a few things that are well worth trying in order to get her started. Kissing her with an ice cube in your mouth just might send shivers all over her. We also recommend using a vibrator like the Lelo Lily, which is great for using on the entire body and will have her purring like a kitten. Take notes in order to build an effective knowledge base on your partner, so that you can move towards more intense and pleasurable experiences.

Creating a Watson

Watsons are an example of intrinsic sexual muscle memory that is attached to a self-perpetuated concept of pleasurable sexual stimulation. What does all that mean? Don't worry, I'm way ahead of you.

Suppose your partner strokes your inner thighs each time after you have an orgasm. These strokes may cause particular associations in your mind, and your inner thighs will become your Watson: an autoerotic erogenous zone. Touching them will turn you on immediately, which is now a conditioned response.

Creating A Watson is the real key in creating a win/win in your sexual relationship. In order to create a Watson, you MUST know how your partner likes to be touched, so that you can create the link between the pleasurable touch that she loves and that thing you love to do.

It also gives you a fail-safe means of turning your partner on. In fact, she likely will find herself placing your hand there as an indicator that she is ready to go! What is better than that?

There is no Watson without Sherlock. So use your Sherlocking skills, build a knowledge base and create a true repertoire with your partner that cannot be duplicated as you are at that point interwoven into her projections of pleasure. No one will know how to touch her in that spot like you. You're the original – the architect – and therefore, become the standard.

Thus, Sherlocking is an indispensable part of the sexual process. It's something you should master before getting into the real act. Without having mastered the craft of Sherlocking, you can never be your most effective in the real act. It's obvious as you can never do well in a field in which you don't know the basic things. This course will be greatly helpful to you in mastering the art of moving ahead with correct steps so that you hit the right target at the right moment. In this way, you will act like a master of the sexual act and not as an inexperienced, desperate and permanent novice just happy to be involved.

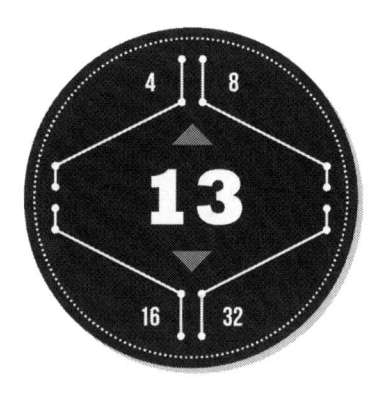

KNOW THY SELF

The better you know yourself, the better your relationship with the rest of the world. - Toni Collette

Let me explain something that is very important. Once you are inside of a woman, it is no longer about the way you look, it's all about the way that you feel. When you get in your feelings, when you become distraught, frustrated or intimidated because of the fact that you hear a woman talking about needing specific sizes, specific looks, specific colors, whatever it may be, consider this: As far as it comes to sex, you have to know that she is giving you a blueprint. She is giving you a blueprint for what she truly wants. You just have to be able to look into what she's saying. Let me explain.

If a woman says she likes girth, if she says she likes a thick cock, what she's really saying is that she likes strokes that stretch. If she says that she likes length, if she says she likes long cocks, she's really saying that she likes strokes that scoop. Now, let's say that she says she likes shallow, she likes average to smaller size cocks. She's saying that clitoral stimulation is truly the thing that turns her on. Now, what if she says she likes it slow. When a woman says she likes it slow, what she's telling you is that she has a very sensitive vagina. What if she says she likes it fast? Well, in that case, she's telling you that she likes heat producing strokes. And what about hard? If a woman says she's like that hard hitting action, what she's saying is that she likes vibration or vibrating strokes.

Do you see that? Do you see how you take that information and make it work for you? You just choose strokes that go with that exact sensation that she wants and then go to work. It's that simple. Just remember, when a woman says that she wants a certain type of penis, she's just telling you that she wants a certain feeling, a feeling that you now can provide. You can do this regardless of your dimensions, you just have to understand one key thing. Sex is internal massage and strokes are internal massage techniques.

Imagine what you could have been if you had known this earlier! Makes you want to catch up to an ex and let her know what she really missed. This can have you feeling like a brand new person, a brand new man with confidence that shifts energy when you enter a room. Once you're inside of her, the only thing that matters is how you feel. Instead of worrying, you lounge in effortless cool. That nagging need to measure yourself against other men, that need that was drilled into you as a natural masculine impulse will be seen as the fear-based reaction it is. That's no longer your condition. Your uniqueness makes doing so allows you to recognize how outright silly and draining it is.

Instead of being apprehensive about going after the women that you truly want, you approach as if it was destined to be. As long as you keep communication open and understand what she wants to feel, match the feelings that she wants to the strokes that give those feelings, you are her prototype. Again, all you need is the strokes and the body that can perform them for synergy.

synergy

noun

1. the interaction or cooperation of two or more organizations, substances, or other agents to produce a combined effect greater than the sum of their separate effects.

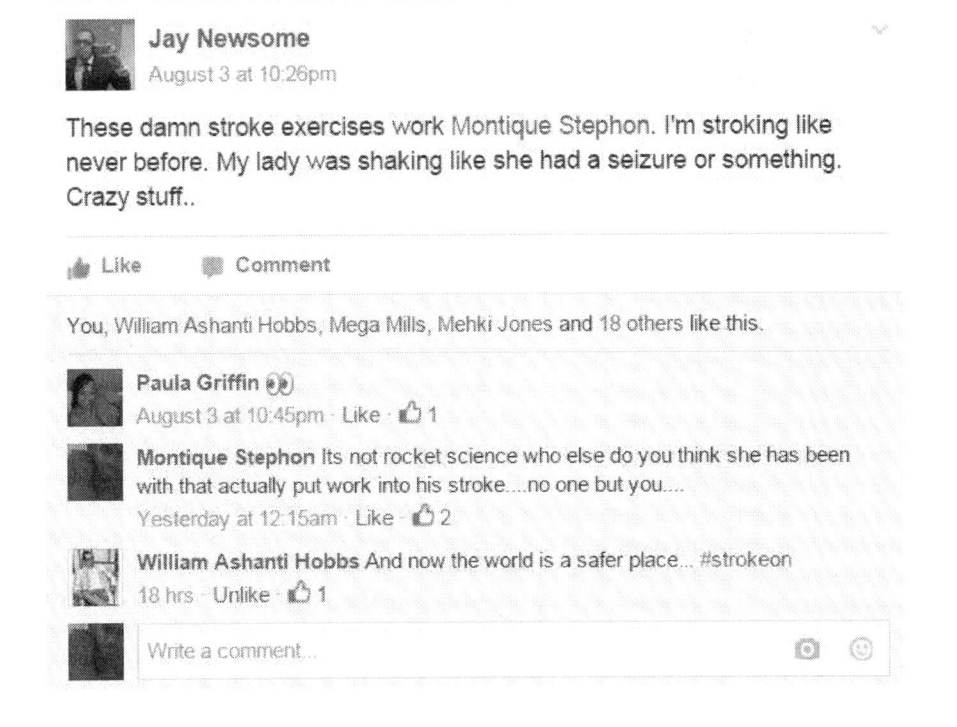

Jay Newsome
August 3 at 10:26pm

These damn stroke exercises work Montique Stephon. I'm stroking like never before. My lady was shaking like she had a seizure or something. Crazy stuff..

👍 Like   💬 Comment

You, William Ashanti Hobbs, Mega Mills, Mehki Jones and 18 others like this.

Paula Griffin 👀
August 3 at 10:45pm · Like · 👍 1

Montique Stephon Its not rocket science who else do you think she has been with that actually put work into his stroke....no one but you....
Yesterday at 12:15am · Like · 👍 2

William Ashanti Hobbs And now the world is a safer place... #strokeon
18 hrs · Unlike · 👍 1

Write a comment...

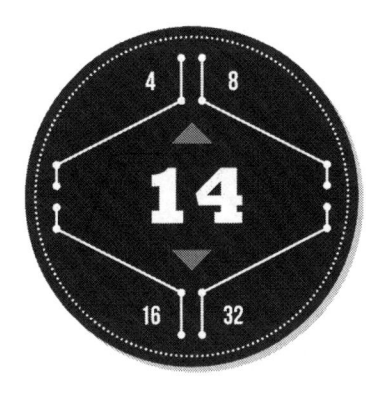

THE AUTO ANGLE

A figure with curves always offers a lot of interesting angles.
- *Wesley Ruggles*

Your concern about your size is warranted. According to a new study in *The Journal of Sexual Medicine,* one-third of women who frequently have vaginal orgasms claim they're more likely to climax when having sex with men with larger penises.

Researchers asked more than 300 women how often they had sex, how frequently they had vaginal and/or clitoral orgasms, and whether or not penis length influenced their ability to orgasm during intercourse. Out of the 160 women who often experienced vaginal-only orgasms and had enough partners to compare sizes, one third said they preferred larger-than-average penises.

So yes, your concern about your size is justified. But ask yourself this: is your interest in pleasing women the reason you want a larger size? If so, taking the pills, having surgeries and buying the products might not solve your concern. Imagine spending tons of your hard-earned money and time to get a few inches larger then realizing that it did nothing for addressing the underlying purpose. If you want to have the kind of size that impacts women, it's all about understanding what *about* size makes a woman climax and using that knowledge to put it to work for yourself.

Vaginal orgasms are often attributed to men finding and stimulating their partner's G-spot, but more recently scientists are finding that the G-spot is really just an extension of the clitoris, and is actually the thing responsible for vaginal orgasms. Two doctors, Dr. Buisson and Dr. Fold, have studied vaginal orgasms in women and have attributed vaginal orgasms to the size, shape and location of the clitoris. The clitoris is larger than it looks; what you see is only the tip of the clitoral iceberg. Their work proved that the clitoris is actually shaped like an inverted wishbone, with just the head of the clitoris and the hood being visible and the rest of the clitoris extending down into the body on either side of the vagina:

Urologist Helen O'Connell of the Royal Melbourne Hospital set out to better understand the microscopic nerve supply to the clitoris using MRI, something that had already been done for men with regard to their sexual function in the 1970s. In 1998 she published her findings, informing the medical world of the true scope and size of the clitoris. Yet ironically that same year, men in America began popping Viagra to cure erectile dysfunction.

In 2005 The American Urological Association published one of Dr. O'Connell's reports on clitoral anatomy. The report itself even states, "The anatomy of the clitoris has not been stable with time as would be expected. To a major extent its study has been dominated by social factors ... Some recent anatomy textbooks omit a description of the clitoris. By comparison, pages are devoted to penile anatomy." The report also mentions how seemingly impossible it is to understand the internal structure of the clitoris with just one diagram. Several are required to truly get a comprehensive understanding of it.

Alas it wasn't until as recent as 2009, French researchers Dr. Odile Buisson and Dr. Pierre Foldès gave the medical world its first complete 3-D sonography of the stimulated clitoris. They did this work for three years without any proper funding. Thanks to them, we now understand how the erectile tissue of the clitoris engorges and surrounds the vagina—a complete breakthrough that explains how what we once considered to be a vaginal orgasm is actually an internal clitoral orgasm.[8]

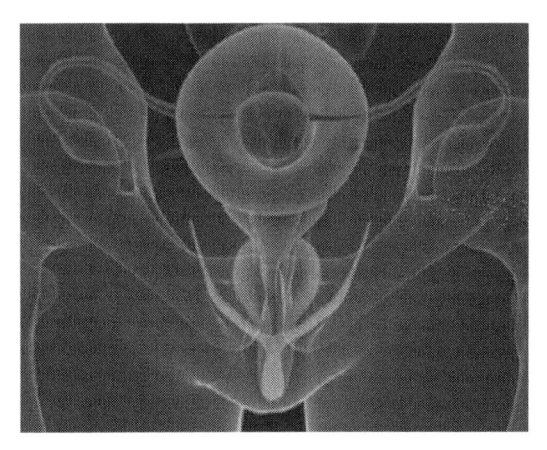

---

8 http://www.museumofsex.com/the-internal-clitoris/

The clitoris is full of nerve endings, roughly 8,000 of them, in fact.[9]

When these nerve endings get stimulated, the clitoris starts to engorge with blood and stiffens. Much of this action happens inside of the body and indeed, the bulk of those nerve endings are in the part of the clitoris that you cannot see. Although you cannot see it, you are engaging it every time she moans and says she wants more. Engaging it is the key to unlocking your partner's ability to have a vaginal orgasm.

We all know that pressure-touch matters when touching and stimulating the clitoris. We know it is sensitive and we need to use certain techniques to ensure that it feels good to her.

Well, just as stimulating the part of clitoris that is visible is important, it is equally important to have techniques to stimulate it internally if we want it to feel good to her.

So your size is applicable in engaging the internal aspects of the clitoris which is buried in the vaginal walls. The issue is the amount in which the internal aspects of the clitoris is buried. This amount varies from woman to woman, so if it is deeply entrenched it helps to have extra girth and length to stimulate it.

That is, however, only when you are *passively* engaging the inner clitoris... With extra girth or size, you have a better chance of stimulating it by accident. But because 99.9% of men don't know that, so many of them fail at making women climax which is why than

---

9   Ibid

more than two thirds (60% of those surveyed) said a larger size made little difference. And once again, why? Because the majority of them, like the rest of us, are engaging the inner clitoris *by accident.*

So what happens when you are purposefully, actively and strategically stimulating it with the knowledge that it is responsible for her orgasm? It is more than possible and will completely remedy any issues you have about size. You have the key, the missing link and the solution for making any woman love you just how you are.

Just as pressure and stroke type matters for stimulating the part of clitoris that is visible, it is equally important to stimulate it internally, using Stroke Skills

When you tilt, turn, twist and encircle her giving her deep clitoral stimulation you will give her an orgasm unlike any that she has ever experienced. When you engage those hidden nerve sensors hidden inside of her body she will be able to have an internal orgasm. Stroke skills gives you an arsenal of techniques so you can vary your rhythm, vary your movement and observe her responses so you know what she likes. When you use your stroke skills techniques, you have an arsenal of movements and rhythms to reach and stimulate even the deepest parts of her clitoris.

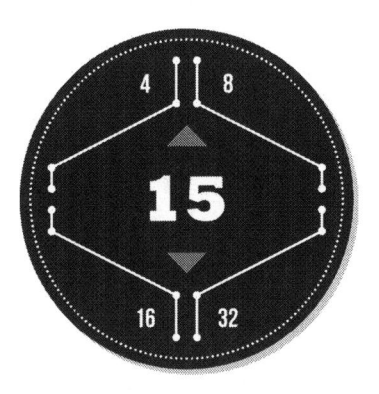

WE JUST HAVE TO CHANGE THE WAY WE THINK

The most useful piece of learning for the uses of life is to unlearn what is untrue. - Antisthenes

A lot of guys today don't have stroke skills, so the question becomes how to deal with the two-strokes that they have: the deep thrust and a shallow thrust. Those are the only strokes that most guys have, so that's what we're going to work with in order to offer a better perspective. How does such an individual create an angle with those two strokes?

Many will opt for doggy-style. The biggest problem with doggy-style is that it is very easy for her to get used to. If you want to wake her up from the back, you have to make your stroke put more pressure on the walls. Too many of us focus on the hole. We focus on the dead space versus what's around the dead space; it's the walls that hold all the sensitivity and response. It's the walls that women feel when you stroke right. It's the sensor in the walls that makes women orgasm, not dead space! That is where your focus needs to be.

This is what you do if you're on your knees hitting it from the back, to create an auto angle you going to take one knee and step that knee forward. You're going to take one knee and step that knee forward and from this point anytime that you stroke your cock is going to go the opposite direction of that knee, any knee that's forward that you put up, the cock is going in opposite direction. In this way when you stroke, it's more like you throwing a hook instead of a jab. Sexologist Giverny Lewis sheds light on that love for a "hook":

A curved penis will push into the walls of the vagina and therefore may feel larger to the woman (as there is more pressure). Depending on which way it bends, it may also stimulate different parts which can increase her pleasure - if it curves upwards towards your stomach you may be stimulating her g-spot when you're on top and her anus (through the vaginal wall) if doing her from behind.[10]

This is how come women like dudes with curves so much. You ever heard a woman go on and on about a dude with a curve in his cock? It's because a guy with a curve has an automatic angle. The problem is you can only throw the hook in one direction so women get used to that, too. You want to change it up. You want to be able to throw angles to the left and you want angles to the right. It's even better if you actually add some real strokes into your arsenal so that you can

---
10 https://www.quora.com/What-is-the-effect-of-a-curved-penis-on-sex

really do some damage angle-wise. But even if you're comfortable sticking with the two-stroke that you know, this will make them more potent. From there, if and when you decide to elevate, you can throw combinations, you can throw a jab, jab hook, you can throw a hook, hook jab… you can come with an uppercut, some over-the-top. Deal with what you have right now and then later, when you're ready to upgrade and when you're ready to put some strokes into your arsenal, visit me at www.strokeskills.com.

From there, you can download the unique strokes and talk about what they do going in and talk about what they do inside of her. I perform them on a live model so that you can see what the position is like. You can see what the rhythm is like and you can see how I'd use them in conjunction with her body, because again, when she's moving you've got to make that stroke modify to it.

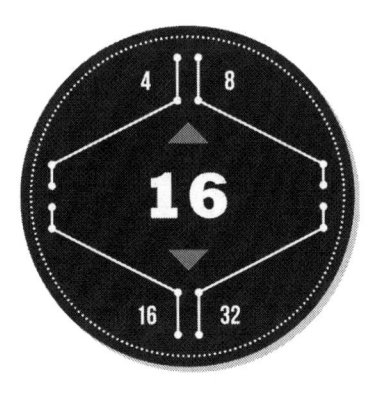

FOCUS VS FORCE

Concentrate all your thoughts upon the work at hand. The sun's rays do not burn until brought to a focus. - Alexander Graham Bell

You have to understand, as a man it is your attention to detail that is going to either make you an incredible lover or a lackluster lover. Your focus is the driving force behind your performance. Knowing how to focus and knowing what to focus on is key.

A lot of you are focusing on the wrong thing. You are starting out going into sex just looking at her vagina. You are looking at the stroke, at going in and out of her. In her mind, she looks at you as being disconnected from the whole process. She starts to thinking, "He is not into me" and her vagina turns off. It gets dry and then she is ready to stop. The only way that you are going to be able to beat something like that happening is if you know what to focus on to keep her in the game, as opposed to making her leave the game. If there's one thing that can go awry in sex, it is what we focus on.

"Few things affect our lives more than our faculty of attention. If we can't focus our attention — due to either agitation or dullness — we can't do anything well. We can't study, listen, converse with others, work, play, or even sleep well when our attention is impaired. And for many of us, our attention is impaired much of the time." - *The Attention Revolution Unlocking the Power of the Focused Mind* by B. Alan Wallace

There are four things to focus on that are so important that even if you don't do anything else, you are still in the game. If you understand it, any stroke that you have is going to be more potent. You want to first focus in on her eyes because you want to be able to re-establish a connection. You want to be able to do that because women, when they cum, when they orgasm, it is not really us making them orgasm; they are getting off based upon the type of attention that we are giving them. That allows them to focus on their own pleasure. That is when she can focus in on what your stroke is doing; that is what makes a woman orgasm. Looking into her eyes is really simple. If she believes that you are there for her and interested in her own pleasure, it allows her to relax. With that relaxation, she can then focus on what you are doing and she can focus on how you are making her feel. That motivates her body to have that orgasm, so focusing in on her eyes is the first thing, and for good reason, according to AJ Harbinger is the CEO and co-founder of The Art of Charm:

S.T.R.O.K.E

To understand why eye contact is so important, we need to appreciate how central it is to the human experience. As it happens, humans — the only primates with white eyes — are drawn to eye contact from an early age. A 2002 study from MIT found that infants were far more likely to try and follow an adult's eyes rather than just their head movements. And beyond the science, think about your personal experience: We study people's eyes to judge their character, we notice when someone meets our gaze, and we are highly conscious of where our eyes wander. Eye contact is deeply rooted in our DNA. In fact, you're reading this article in large part because your caveman ancestors had an intuitive mastery of eye contact. Back then, eye contact meant the difference between life and death, attraction and indifference.[11]

Secondly, you want to be able to focus in on rhythm. When she takes her hands and wraps them around your hips or she reaches back and pulls you into her; it's not because she is trying to instruct your stroke more or less; she is trying to give you a rhythm, she is trying to tell you, "Okay if you stay on this rhythm, I am going to have an orgasm. This rhythm, this style, this pace of massage is pleasurable to me." So you want to play attention to that. Even though we live in a society where we as men tend to lead, in this situation, you want her to set the rhythm and synchronize to that if you want to make her orgasm.

The third and most important thing to pay attention to when you are stroking a woman is something that you probably never thought about: how she is moving her hips. During sex, a woman's hips are almost like the steering wheel for how your cock massages her walls. It

---

11   http://theartofcharm.com/flirting-and-attraction/science-eye-contact-attraction/

doesn't even necessarily matter what you do with your hips and what you do with your stroke because the second she starts moving, she can navigate what you touch inside of her. So, you need to pay attention to where and how she is moving her hips. She is going to push you against the places that are most pleasurable to her, she is going to push you towards her spot. This is a real key in finding a woman's spot. If you pay attention, you don't have to guess. If you pay attention, you are going to know exactly how to move and exactly what walls to stroke, because she is going to push you there. And do you know how you will know when you are on the right wall? When you are using the right stroke, she is going to start breathing heavy and those hips, they are going to stop moving. You will be there, you have arrived.

At that point, that's when you reach into your arsenal of strokes and you start unleashing as many different strokes as you have on that wall until you start to see her clinch up. That is when you want to focus in on the specific stroke that made her do that; that's the one you use, at her pace and at her rhythm.

Now like I said when we started this, you need to stop staring at her vagina when you are stroking, it creates a disconnect with her. If you don't, it's going to turn it off and she is not going to feel all of the things that you are doing. Sex is mental to women, first and foremost. It starts with the mental component. You have to make sure that you check off those mental boxes, those mental areas before the sex is introduced into the situation. It is not that you just suck and therefore she isn't into you. There are scientific reasons for this need for mental stimulation:

Her hormonal funding of testosterone, a hormone in both men and women that governs physiological craving for sex, can be as low as 100th of yours. Think about weightlifting with and without steroids. You can do everything that your buddy does curl for curl, but if he's on steroids his rate of build is going to be much higher. A man's normal testosterone levels are 300-1,000 ng/dL serum blood. Parents of teenage girls are afraid of the 1,000 level, and at 300, a guy often seeks a sex therapist for low desire. At 300, he won't have morning erections, he struggles even with Viagra, will think about sex about once a week, and if he has a fight with his wife he won't want it. A woman's testosterone level is about 70 ng/dL when she is 18 and half that when she is 40 if she's lucky. Her experience in her body is markedly different that your experience. While we may process testosterone differently and there are also measurements that are even more sensitive, this is the primary reason you crave sex and she doesn't. She likes it, she needs it but she only knows that once she's having it.[12]

---

12 https://www.psychologytoday.com/blog/married-and-still-doing-it/201209/five-sex-tips-men-about-women

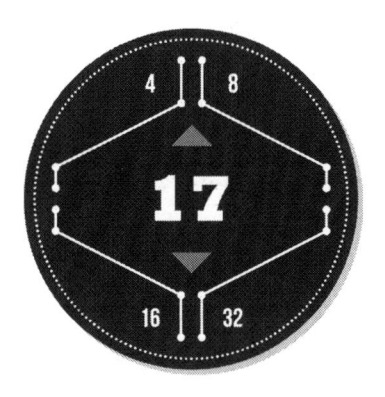

SEXUAL RECALIBRATION

Recalibration of the mind means clearing our perceptions and recovering our capacity for pure observation. — Ilchi Lee

Thanks to technology, we are deluged with media and advertising. Movies are no longer something that must be experienced in the movie theater, and we no longer have to be in front of the TV in our living rooms to watch. We have smart phones, laptops, wireless TV receivers, digital musical players, digital e-book readers, and netbooks and tablets; in short, we are always just a click away from being able to watch something.

We are exposed to media everywhere we go now. For the most part, that can be a good thing. It is good to be able to reach out with a few swipes of a finger and be able to watch a movie on your mobile device. Just browsing the internet, you get pop-up ads aplenty from anything from weight loss to erection aids. Along with portable media, we get portable advertisements. It used to be that product advertisements appeared only on bus stops, billboards, and while watching TV and now, as long as there is the internet, we get ads. We are saturated in media. We go to any website and we see ads.

If you go to any blog, you will find that certain words are linked to ads – we are under a deluge of media and advertising. The media that we see is there to shape our ideals, to guide us into conforming to the ideals of society. However, who decides on what the ideals of society are? The media, that's who! The media does not have our best interests at heart. They are not filling our heads with images and ideals because they are altruistic and want to help us. No. Media is motivated by one thing and one thing only, greed. Think about it. The media floods us with images and how they think we ought to be and we watch it. Unless you go off the grid totally, you cannot escape it.

People in remote areas of Fiji had almost no exposure to television until 1995. That's when their government began allowing TV stations to broadcast Western programs. Almost overnight, youth became exposed to Western media.

Until very recently, Fiji's culture valued large, robust and strong-boned women. In fact, the culture encouraged women to eat a lot. When Becker started looking for evidence of eating disorders in 1995, she couldn't find a single report of a girl in Fiji who had purged — vomited — to manage her weight. Then Western TV exploded onto the scene. People started watching shows such as *Beverly Hills 90210*, *Melrose Place* and *The X-Files*. Becker wondered if the images and ideas in these shows might have affected peoples' views of what the ideal woman should look like.

And sure enough, signs of a change were emerging by 1998. In one small survey of teen girls in Fiji, slightly more than one in every 10 reported having vomited to lose weight. "That is an oh-my-gosh kind of finding," says Becker. "That's about what you would expect in a Massachusetts high school." In addition, more than three-quarters of the girls reported that television influenced their body image. Becker and her colleagues reported the results in a 2002 study[13] in the *British Journal of Psychiatry*.[14]

The media tells us that we must be thin. We see movies with girls so thin that we can count their ribs; actresses show up on the red carpet at events looking so frail, as if a strong wind will carry them away and they are the media darlings. Media does the same thing to us when it comes to sex, intimacy and our very ideals about what is and is not sexy. If every love story has an actress that is a size 0 in it, then men become conditioned to find that size sexy and women who are not a size 0, stand very little chance. However, most women are not a size 0, 2, or even 4! Our own ideas about what is sexy gets drowned out. Women see the media portraying men as tall, muscled, and clean-shaven and just like the women, when we are bombarded with this image; we begin to fixate on it as being a measure of how flawed we are.

---

13 http://www.ncbi.nlm.nih.gov/pubmed/12042229
14 http://www.bbc.com/news/health-29569473

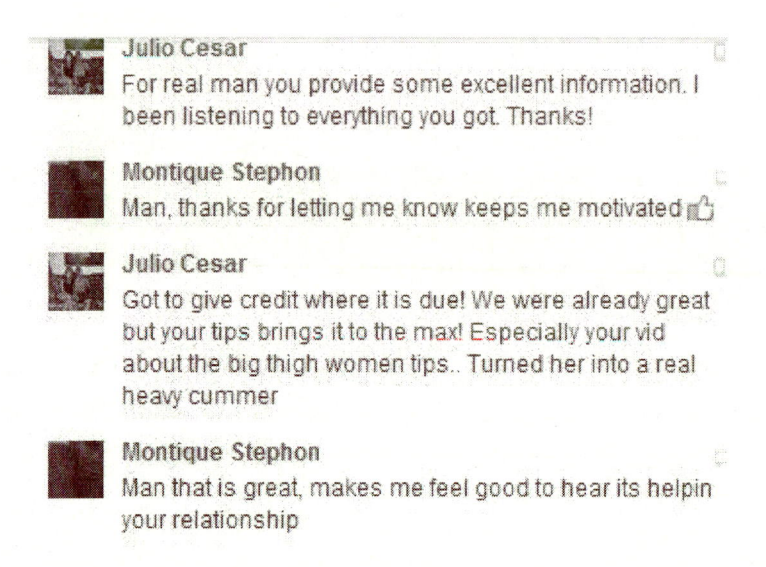

> **Julio Cesar**
> For real man you provide some excellent information. I been listening to everything you got. Thanks!
>
> **Montique Stephon**
> Man, thanks for letting me know keeps me motivated 👍
>
> **Julio Cesar**
> Got to give credit where it is due! We were already great but your tips brings it to the max! Especially your vid about the big thigh women tips.. Turned her into a real heavy cummer
>
> **Montique Stephon**
> Man that is great, makes me feel good to hear its helpin your relationship

We put too much faith in the media; we assume that what the media is showing us is realistic, when in fact it is not. Media is fiction, and we need to stay cognizant of that because fiction can be manipulated. When you allow that fiction to manipulate you, then you are allowing yourself to be changed based on something that is designed solely to make money for others! They tell us that we must have this body type, this hair color, perfect teeth, and that men must possess rippling muscles and powerful, long-lasting erections. They tell us all of this, and then they proceed to shove advertisements for all of these products down our throats and because we want to be "normal," we buy them!

When it comes to sex in the movies, everything seems to center around the act of sex itself. Harder is better and long is the only way to go. The problem with the media's portrayal about sex is just that. In the same way they project unrealistic body images, they showcase sex in an equally unrealistic fashion.

The entire point of sex is that it is produces pleasure. You receive pleasure from another and you enjoy giving it as well. Sex in the media has very little to do with actual pleasure, although the actresses and actors might be very good about acting as if it does. Being a good lover is about more than just hard and fast sex.

Yes, there are those who make sex their profession, but that is not who I am discussing at the moment. This is for the rest of us, the regular people, the average Joes, the guy next door. Even though you might be good at sex, you are still an amateur – we all are! When we are born, we are comfortable with our bodies and with being naked. It is only as we grow up that we are told to cover up, don't touch yourself, don't do this, and don't do that. When it comes to sex, there are a lot more 'don'ts' than there are things that we are told that we should do and that is backwards. Although we are all born with the equipment, there is no manual that gets handed to us when we are old enough to have sex, nothing that tells us how to give or receive pleasure. Knowing the basic mechanics of sex is not enough, but we do not know that since the media has forced all of these unrealistic ideas into our heads.

Sex is mostly trial and error. We are taught how to drive a car, how to ride a bike, and how to do many things, but when it comes to learning about sex, we are mostly left to our own devices. We fumble in the dark, we recall the movies we have seen and try to imitate those, we talk to our friends and compare stories and techniques, but really, we are all amateurs.

Knowing how to have sex is far from knowing how to have sex well. Sex is often nothing more than going on our instincts to put it in and pray that it feels good for both. When the sex is unsatisfying, it begins to erode away our egos. Why can't we please her? Why can't I get her to orgasm when I used to be able to? What am I doing wrong? When you begin to doubt yourself, it will begin to affect your relationship. Lack of confidence can be a relationship killer. It all links back to the fact that we are amateurs and we really have no idea what we are doing when it comes to sex. We say a little prayer and then move about and hope that something magical happens. It is like finding buried treasure with only half a treasure map – you can come close but you will never find the spot.

When it comes to our sexuality, is putting it in and praying good enough? No! Porn shows us a variety of positions, all of which the woman seems to be enjoying, but when you try it at home, you do not get the same results. Going back to when we were young, we were comfortable in our own skin. We had no pre-conceived notions about sex or about how we were expected to perform. When you are comfortable in your own skin, when you are confident, there is nothing sexier than that. That is something that no pill can give you, confidence. It does not matter how big you are or how long you can stay hard; you can learn to be a great lover just as you are. Porn, according to sociologist Marc LaFrance, is most likely at the heart of this "crisis of masculinity":

There's a link to be made between this so-called crisis of masculinity . . . and the extraordinary proliferation of erectile dysfunction products, the rise of body building and cosmetic surgery, the high-energy drinks, and let's throw in for the good measure the boom in grooming products... All of these suggest in my view an increased preoccupation with male bodies in which they're all trying to increase the maleness of the male. Pec implants, calf implants, penile enhancement — these are very aligned with that hegemonic or hyper masculinity. Just as all those female products speak to women's insecurity, these are tapping into a growing anxiety around masculinity and an alpha male ideal.[15]

Think of sex as an internal massage when you watch porn, and you will notice a lot of thrusting. In fact, you will see almost nothing but thrusting in and out. The majority of porn focuses on a woman being in position and then having the guy thrust into her repeatedly. For porn stars, they are performing for the camera, but for the rest of us, we are performing for the woman that we are with. So, why mimic the moves that we see in porn if they do not bring any pleasure? Because we do not know any different! That is why! Stop thinking of sex like a machine, with a piston that bangs in and out and think of sex in terms of a massage; an internal massage. With sex, you are trying to please her inside and out, just like you were giving her an internal massage. Erase what you have learned from porn from your mind.

> Wachena Woodard Amen to that!!! Most guys don't even have a clue and when you tell them about stroke skills they turn up their noses.. like joker here is the key here sometimes you have to apply yourself.. I love when a guy do something that I'm not use to.. because men tend to go in patterns and stick to that one said pattern... you have to switch it up.. I love being caught off guard with something new like wow you didn't do that the last time.. wonder what else you have in your pockets like the fun intimacy begin. 😊
> 18 mins · Unlike · 👍 1

---

15 http://www.montrealgazette.com/health/does+porn+make+males+insecure+about+bodies/6067786/story.html

The actual vaginal opening is not where all of her pleasure comes from, so continuing to enter her, then pull out, and then enter her again rapidly is a media trick. It is shot that way to showcase the act of penetration only. Remember, those are actors, they get paid to "enjoy" it. The pleasure from sexual intercourse does not come from penetration. Instead of focusing on the vaginal opening; shift your attention to the walls of the vagina instead. When you are having sex with the intention of simply going in and out rapidly, you are missing all of her hot spots, the vaginal walls. What makes sex sensual for a woman is the sensation of friction and pressure on the vaginal walls, it is not about how deep you can go, or if you can hit her cervix, it is about how many internal spots you can hit while having sex. By positioning yourself so as you move, you are hitting her vaginal walls; that's what builds up the friction and pleasure, ending in an orgasm. There is a misconception that says that it is near impossible to give your partner an orgasm through penetration alone.

It is impossible to give her an orgasm through penetration if you do not know what you are doing, that much is true! However, by using yourself to massage the inner walls of her vagina, you can produce a slow buildup of pleasure, bringing her deliciously closer to ecstasy until she finally orgasms. When we learn from the movies, we learn all of the wrong things! This is why a sexual re-calibration is necessary if you want to be a good lover. Going straight in and out might bring you to orgasm, but it does nothing for her. Sex is about intimacy and pleasure. Sex is a give and take situation, not only do you get pleasure but you give it as well and so you owe it to your partner to know how to pleasure her. Once you do, your relationship will soar to new heights, along with your pleasure and hers. Every motion that you make has the possibility of being sensual, of feeling good, and of building up that sexual tension that explodes into an orgasm for her. Sex is a full-body experience and when you go into with that mindset, everything is sensual and everything will feel good, for both of you. When you are making every move count by hitting the vaginal walls in all of the right ways, things like size no longer matter.

Guys are so hung up on their size that they forget that it has very little to do with size and a whole lot to do with technique. As you enter her, you are massaging her in the most intimate of ways, engaging in sensations that she will love! The question becomes, how do you know how to use sex as an internal massage when the movies all focus on sex in all of the wrong ways? The answer falls once again on Zenity Fitness, or to be exact, their Stroke Skills program. Stroke skills is a kinetic exercise program for men, not only will it tone you but it will give you increased stamina, endurance, and flexibility; allowing you to be a better lover. This unique program will not only train you to perform better, but it will make you more fit as well. The exercises in this program are optimal for teaching you techniques and movements that will allow you to truly be massaging the walls of her vagina, bringing her nothing but pleasure.

The exercises taught to you in this program are all designed to engage the muscle groups used during sex, meaning not only will you get all of the health benefits from exercise but your sex life will soar. S.T.R.O.K.E. stands for systematic, tactile, rhythmically, organized, kinetic, exercises and that is an apt description for the exercises set, which use your own body weight to strengthen and tone. This combination of core strengthening exercises and movements translate very well for the bedroom, increasing your ability and your confidence. The rhythmic nature of the exercises is designed to heighten and expand your sexual experiences, so that you will be truly working on pleasuring your partner, from the inside out. You can do the exercises alone, or for a deeply intimate encounter, with your partner.

> Isaac T. Johnson Man I used to have a gut and after like 3 months of stroke skills, my body toned up. And yes that shit does work in the bedroom
> May 24 at 2:44am · Unlike · 👍 1

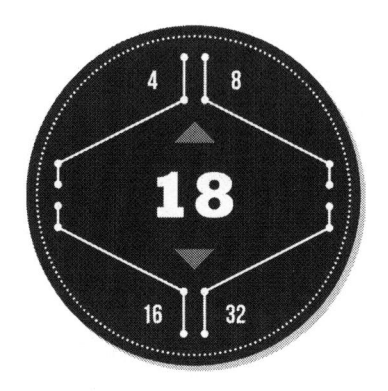

HURRY UP AND BANG

To study the abnormal is the best way of understanding the normal.
- William James

We live in a fast-paced world. People want everything now, and they do not want to wait. We have fast food, apps at our fingertips and a houseful of gadgets that are supposed to make our lives easier. However, there is one thing where quicker is not better and that is when it comes to sex! Media has misguided us all again, from blockbuster movies to porn, sex is always something done hard and fast and both parties are always satisfied. Now, is there a time and a place for a quickie every now and then? Of course! But not every time. Foreplay is all but nonexistent in the media's eyes. A few frantic kisses, some groping, perhaps a few seconds of cunnilingus but then straight to hard and fast penetration. No matter what position, the sex is hard and fast. Sex is not a race, and you get no grand prize for finishing first. Once again, the media is leading us astray from how to actually pleasure a woman. If everybody only did what they saw in the movies, orgasms would be a rare thing indeed.

When you are in the heat of passion is there an increase in the rhythm? Naturally, of course there is. However, the media wants us to believe that from start to finish, it should be hard and fast. Repeatedly slamming into her can cause her pain, and the repeated hard motion and the friction that it causes is far from the sensual type. In fact, sex that way will actually numb the vagina and means that she gets no benefit from the sexual act. And, very often, this type of sex is painful. Her ability to achieve orgasm has nothing to do with how hard you penetrate her, or how franticly you pump your hips. Her ability to achieve orgasm has everything to do with you making sex a full body encounter, taking your time, and building up to one or more orgasms for you both.

Take the veil off of your eyes that the media has placed there, and learn to experience sex as it is meant to be: a sensual and tantalizing experience for you both. Sex should be savored and enjoyed. The media teaches men that the faster they go, the more passionate they must feel and so they feel that in order to prove that they are passionate about their partner, they feel that they must mimic what the media tells us, that passion equals hard and fast.

Trust us, your partner does not equate hard and fast with passion, because that type of sex is most definitely not pleasurable to her and passion is about feeling good. If you make her feel good, then she knows that you are passionate about her! It has nothing to do with having just enough foreplay to get her wet and then entering her, slamming into her until you are done and then calling it a great sex session. The media, again, has it totally backwards. Passion is when you evoke all of the senses – you taste her, you touch her, you see her, you hear her, and you smell her. You want to enjoy her when you have sex, which is passion. When you dedicate yourself to her pleasure, *that* is passion. When you take your time to focus every part of her body and you make the sex count (not simply mechanical in-and-out sex), *that* is passion. You will not see that in the media though, and that is exactly why the media is unreliable as a source for sex.

The media tells us what they want us to learn, because they can capitalize on it somehow. Our needs are not important to them, but earning money is. And yet we continue to let the media guide us and influence us when it comes to sex and sensuality. Pleasuring your partner takes skill and patience, and there is no skill to what the media tells us is passionate sex. In reality, sex starts with a touch, a kiss, or even a look. It begins before clothes come off and it is a time to slowly explore your partner, with your hands, your mouth, and your body. Why rush it and turn a good thing into something that is merely so-so for you and uneventful for her? In fact, face any clocks in the room towards the wall because there is no 'hurry up' when it comes to good sex. Good sex takes as long as it needs to or wants to. Every part of you will be dedicated to pleasing her, and the response that you get from her when you take your time like that will be like none you have ever seen. There is no ego booster in the world like leaving your partner exhausted, weak-kneed, and happy. Your confidence will go up and your relationship will go to new levels.

When done right and when done slow, sex is a chance to connect to your partner, which is beneficial to relationships. There is no connection when the sex is hard and fast, despite what the media says. The encounter is so brief and is so devoid of passion that no connection (other than the brief physical connection) is made. Real people know that the passion lies within the *way* you have sex, not in how fast. Take your time and appreciate her every curve, massage her, massage her internally as you have sex, with deliberate movements that press against the vaginal walls, pleasure her orally, but engage all of the senses for a deeply satisfying sexual encounter for your both. When you take it slow your partner can appreciate your skills, because the experience will be vastly different from the media portrayal of "wham-bam-thank-you-ma'am" sex.

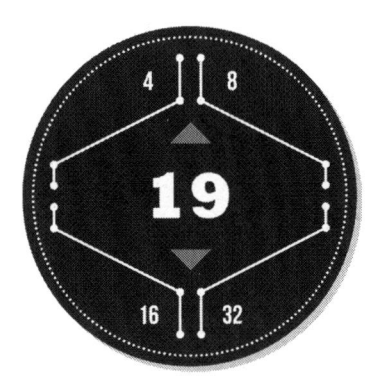

YOUR END IS HER BEGINNING

It's easier to resist at the beginning than at the end.
- Leonardo da Vinci

It happens over and over again in the movies and on the shows that we watch on TV: sex is over when the man has his orgasm. He then rolls off and goes to sleep or goes back to doing whatever he had been doing before. Because of this, men tend to end sex after they come, figuring that since they came, it is over. Media tells us that this is acceptable and that it is just how things are done. It is *not* how it is done! It is another manipulation of us by the media.

Sex is not over just because the male partner comes. It does not trigger the end credits or signal the end of anything, unless you want it to. Why would you want it to end there? Sex feels good, correct? When you pleasure your partner, it makes you feel confident and sexy, correct?

So why would you choose to end sex at what is actually a very good launch point for an even better session of sensual and pleasing sex? Because of the refractory period, men tend to think that since it takes them awhile to be able to get erect again, that it means that sex is over.

Wrong! You should be using that refractory period to heighten her pleasure and seeing her writhing about in ecstasy. It's excellent visual stimulation to help shorten that refractory period down. Your orgasm is just the beginning of hers. Chances are that she may not have even had an orgasm before you have, so this is your chance to keep her going, to use your fingers and mouth to bring her to the brink and ecstasy and then right over the edge to orgasms. Additionally, many women are capable of having multiple orgasms. They might not even know that they are capable of this, because nobody has ever taken the time to see if they are. And even if they are not, it will still be a pleasurable experience for you both because even if she only has one orgasm, it will be toe-curling fantastic for her.

Chances are, with foreplay, sex and followed by your continued attention, you can tease multiple orgasms from her. With each orgasm, they get stronger and stronger, so the more she has, the pleasure she feels increases exponentially. Ignore the media; when you ejaculate, it is the start of a new phase in your lovemaking. Instead of ending the session and opting to take a nap while she is unhappy and unfulfilled, you can make sure that her needs are not only met but that they are exceeded. Use your refractory period to continue to tease and please her, so that she has already had at least one and hopefully multiple orgasms by the time that you are fully recharged and ready to go.

Sex is so much more than just the act itself, and a man who understands and follows this line of thinking will have a very happy partner indeed. As mentioned before, sex is about engaging every sense for you both so when you need to recharge your batteries (so to speak), you can use your fingers on her, inside and out, and your mouth. You have more tools at your disposal than just your penis, so keep them all in mind. Do not let her cool down just because you need to recharge. You can skillfully keep her motor running, bringing to heights of pleasure that will only go higher and higher. The connection between the two of you will be like nothing else, because since you have already had an orgasm you will be fully focused on her and only her.

That is passion. By focusing on her after you have come, you will be turning good sex into fantastic sex. Pleasing her increases your confidence, it makes you feel good, and it helps the two of you connect. There is no excuse for not taking every opportunity to please her fully and that is why your end is her beginning. You may have 'finished,' but you are far from finished.

The problem is, that oral sex and manual manipulation by using your fingers can be just as hit or miss as actual sex because once again, there is nothing to tell us, "hey do this to make her feel great!" Oral sex and using your fingers is just glossed over in porn, and once again, what they do show is not done for pleasure, it is to allow for the best camera angle only. Do not rely on what you see to help you be a great lover when it comes to using your mouth and finger. You can become a master at oral sex through another of Zenity Fitness's programs. Zynergistics.com is the program that teaches you how to use your mouth and hands to pleasure your partner.

Oral sex is about much more than just placing your mouth on her and then flicking your tongue around, if you do not know where and how to use your tongue, you are left floundering, and just as you hit the right spot, and you lose it again! Zynergistics will train you to not only find the G-spot, but how to massage it to give her a powerful orgasm, unlike any other. It will also teach you how to be a master at cunnilingus and using your fingers to bring her to orgasm.

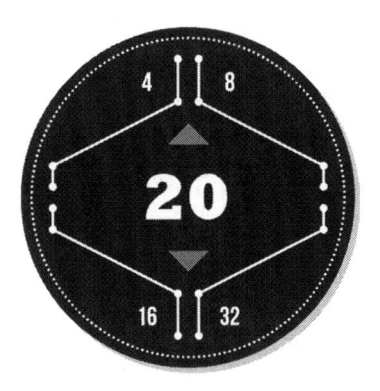

EXIT STROKING

Affairs are easier of entrance than of exit; and it is but common prudence to see our way out before we venture in. - Aesop

What's the sweet spot? No it's not the clitoris, no it's not the G spot – it has nothing to do with those things. The sweet spot is that exit stroke. (Once again, for all of you who don't know, when you stroke into a woman, you have the in stroke and that's when you go in and you have the exit stroke and that's when you come out. Your in-stroke and your exit stroke should both be different because you want to engage different parts of her walls going in and coming out.

Women win on the front-end, men win on the back-end. – Patrice O'Neal

Keeping a woman on her toes is best, so we don't like them to always know what we're going to do so that they can brace for it and not get the full impact. You want to make sure your exit stroke is on an angle and you want to drag on the exit. Stroke in, pause or stop and when you come out you're going to drag on an angle. Take that wall with you because if you don't do this the most important part of the stroke is being missed. When you train your stroke skills, I want you to practice the exit stroke. I want you to practice one stroke going in and doing a completely different stroke coming out. I want you get used to that because when you can do that you will be able to find out that a lot of times after you stroke in a woman changes her position. She either might roll her hips, she might scoop you or she might scoop down, so the spot to engage has moved, understand?

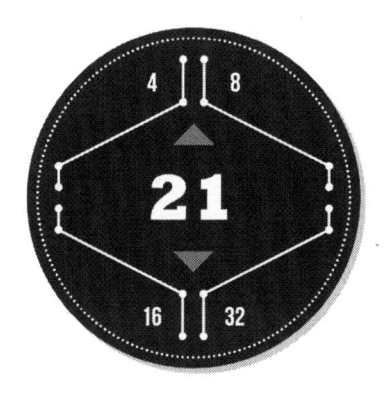

STROKE FREQUENCY

If you want to find the secrets of the universe, think in terms of energy, frequency and vibration. — Nikola Tesla

How long does it take for a woman to pick up on your stroke change? Good question. Let's take it back to basics. We all know that a stroke is an artistic way of moving in and out of a woman while focusing on massaging her walls. We are looking at sex as a massage; ultimately a woman will orgasm if the massage is good. Remember, strokes are internal massage techniques. It takes a woman a second to recognize when your stroke changes.

Now why is that important? As stated earlier, when you are stroking inside of a woman, you are paying attention to what the different massages do – but you have to use each massage long enough to figure if it is the right one for her. She is not going to start 'ooing and aahing' right off the bat. She is going to have to take some time and feel you and if she feels you and it feels right, she is going to give you that cue, that 'ooo' that 'aww.' She is going to clamp down on you giving you and indicator that 'yes, this feels fantastic.' So you want to keep using it, but if you go in there and you are moving too fast or you are using too many strokes that are right behind each other in too quick of a succession, she won't get a chance to truly feel you and to recognize your skill.

This is why when you are stroking, you want to deliver at least 10 strokes fast or 5 strokes slow before you move to the next strokes. This is just so you can get her to feel you and give you some type of indication if this is the one or if you want to keep moving to different strokes.

Some men have invested heavily in stroke skills and have mastered 10-15 different strokes and we always want to use different ones because they feel good on our cock and it's fun to be able to see how see responds to them, however we have to remember that we are inside of this woman and she can feel what we are doing. If we are moving through our stuff too quick or if we are not giving her a chance to feel it, this will dry her up. When you do these strokes too fast and you are pulling out of her too quick, you are taking the moisture that's inside and you are drawing the moisture out. I must reiterate, if you are pulling the wetness out of her body if you are moving too fast and there is nothing wrong with moving too fast, once you have a stroke that see likes and once you know that she wants it fast like that. But if you are immediately moving at a rapid pace, when you start stroking what it is going to do is it's going to keep her from being able to tell if she can enjoy that stroke. Is that clear?

It's going to take at least 5 slow or 10 fast, so that she can tell if this is a stroke that she wants you to move with or if you should continue strolling through your catalogue for the one that is going to knock it out of the park.

Nick Mack   10:29am
Yo! I made her orgasm in less than 30 seconds.. just by z stroking. That's it. I hadn't even gotten into my routine. She said she'd never felt anything like that before.

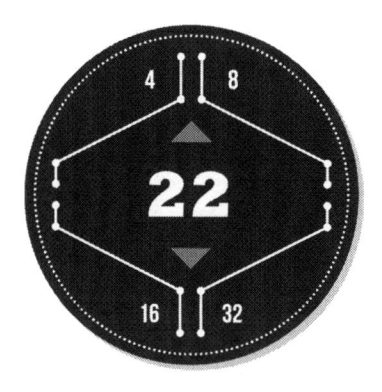

INFLECTION & MISDIRECTION

Our minds have a tendency to wander. To duck and feint and keep us at a slight remove from the moment at hand. - Dani Shapiro

Audio and rhythm are very important areas of your sexual physique. They are areas that you have to work on and if you do so, will increase your capacity to please your lover for longer and with a more exciting style than ever before. The main reason is that your ability to be audio tuned, to be synced up to your audio, gives you the capacity to create your own style.

The difference between styles is a person's ability to add their own special sauce into it. Yes, time for you to be an artist. You don't want to have a style like me. Sure you might like my stroke style, however you want to have a style that is connected to you. You want to make sure that is representative of your own flavor because you want to get a woman hooked on you. Not on Montique, on you.

So the more things that you can do to incorporate your own flavor, the more that women will be wanting your unique strokes and the sensations that only you can bring them. It's going to make you feel more grounded in your sexuality, in your masculinity and in your confidence.

So all that being said, audio and rhythm creates unique styles. I want to talk to you about three different areas of inflection; audio inflection. Now what is audio inflection? Audio inflection is basically the concept that you can accentuate your stroke through changing the rhythm of your stroke. There are three different ways that you can accentuate your stroke.

Stroke volume is the intensity that you are using a stroke. I am not talking about speed; I am talking about intensity; how much pressure are you applying your stroke? The more pressure, the more volume.

So you might be doing a regular stroke on this beat and then you add inflection. So after doing one stroke and then you turn the volume up on one stroke that you think she really enjoys, so that she feels it a little bit more. On the same situation, you can do something were you actually turn it down and when you turn a volume down on a stroke, often it's going to be for misdirection. Let's say we are throwing a good five strokes:

beat, beat, beat, beat, *low beat*, beat.

You see that? Did you see how on the fifth beat I did not use the same amount of pressure?

So what it did is that she could not react or expect the stroke the same way. So the last one that hit, the number 5, I make that on harder and see really feels it; because you see women subconsciously will expect the stroke; they are rhythmic beings, women do everything on rhythm. They orgasm on rhythm and their cycle happens on a rhythm; they are organically rhythmic. So when they have sex, a woman will naturally tune in to your beat. So when you stroke regular like most of us do; being 1,2,3,4 or faster 1234, she is going to modify her body so that see reacts to that stroke in a way that is pleasing to her or that see believes is pleasing to her. But sometimes they do it out of fear and it kind of keeps their orgasm bottled up.

A woman sometimes can predict your stroke. When she braces for the stroke and you deliver it, your stroke is dampened. It does not have the authority that it would have had if she had accepted it with complete receptivity. Therefore, when you do something like set a misdirection, when you turn down the volume on your stroke when she sees things it is going to be turned up, it confuses her. When her rhythm is confused, that is when you can stroke with a stroke and really make her feel it. I will do it again. (beat, beat, beat, beat, soft beat, beat) Got it?

Now these are a couple of techniques that you can add to your stroke skills to truly turn up the effects of your unique style and by that I mean; you need to make sure that she can recognize your style; you need to make her recognize what you can do like no other.

So you are not going to use the average in and out pull stick strokes.

You can still use them sometimes bros but listen, you want to use strokes skills; you want to find some stroke skills that you can be expert with because you have to know, nobody knows these but you. You are like 1 in a billion people if you know some stroke skills. So you have to understand that when you use these on a woman, they set in some muscle memory that is going to make her remember you. When you use that stroke with a specific signature style, like either turning up the volume or missing a step, using misstep/misdirection, that is something that she is going to learn to love and respect and that she will know she can find no place else.

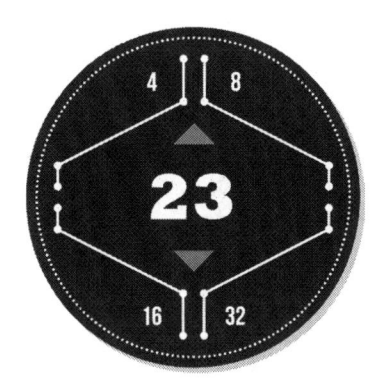

STUTTER STROKING

I've been in relationships before where my girl intentionally wouldn't tell me know how good I was because she didn't want me to get cocky and be out in the streets. This is a psychological thing: it's the same reason why if you are really good, they won't tell their friends. They are not going to tell their friends if they you really have skills. They are going to keep that to themselves and they will give you a really mean look if their girlfriends come over and you just happen to be in your boxers practicing your stroke skills with the door open. It is what it is.

In any event this is the situation; if you are dealing with a girl like mine who often would not want to let me know when I was really putting that good work in, you have to do something called adding a stutter to your stroke; da-da-da that's right, you are adding a stutter to your stroke. What that does is throw a woman off from being able to pick up your rhythm. Let me tell you what that means. The way that women can dampen the effect of your stroke is that your stroke for most of you is the same one over and over and over again. They know how to move and arch so when you really should be hitting a spot and sending some serious pleasure up into the yoni, instead they dampen it so you don't hit that spot. In fact, they know how to move so you don't even get a full stroke in. It is because they know how to read your rhythm. They have caught your rhythm.

Now a lot of you all don't have stroke skills. A lot of you all only have two strokes in your arsenal; you got a short stroke and you got a long stroke, that's all you have; so she knows what to expect from you. I am just going to be real with you, she knows what you are going to bring and she doesn't want you putting your dick in her heart, making her all dick-matized, which is defined as, courtesy of singer Jill Scott:

"Where you get caught up in the whole sexuality of your relationship but it's not going anywhere... Just somebody giving you the goods but not necessarily giving you the rest-or not expecting the rest from them."[16]

She wants to stay very indifferent about your skills. It's real. She wants to feel like, "Ahh, I can take it or leave it." She doesn't want to start going through withdrawal about you and is sabotaging your stroke to make that happen. To hell with that. You're a good dude and good dudes shouldn't have to suffer. I am going to tell you how to take it all back. And like I said, it is about a-add-adding a stutter to your stroke.

You can liken a stutter to a crossover; it has the same concept. The

---

16 http://www.clutchmagonline.com/2011/07/oh-word-jill-scott-says-she-was-dickmatized-can-you-relate/

S.T.R.O.K.E

idea is to have her think that you are going to go one way and you go the opposite direction or you are going to stick were you are; in fact, that's the one that really catches them when you stick. You are going to actually do a stroke, stroke out, do a stroke, stroke out again and on the third stroke you are going to go quarter in... then stroke out and then back in really quick again.

So rhythmically it is going to be like this, "tap, tap, tap, tap tap tap." Now when you add the stutter right after it, right there is going to be a point where she is completely open, because see you caught her slipping and at that point her guard came down and the chocha is fully receptive. That is where you throw your best stroke in. Unfortunately for many of you, you only have two so best your stroke is either going be your long stroke or your short stroke. For those of you were smart enough to get stroke skills, you can throw a Latin stroke in there, you can throw a Bachata stroke in there, you can throw a U stroke, you can throw a shocker, you can throw tons of different things and get that spot.

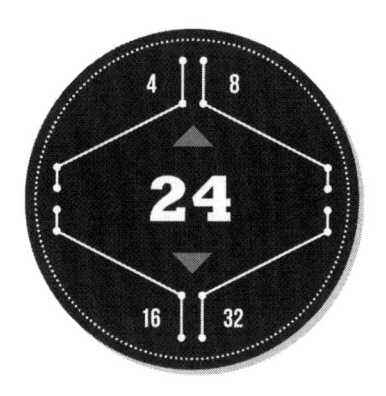

RAW GUY TALK; SIT INTO YOUR STROKE

It is because the body is a machine that education is possible. Education is the formation of habits, a super inducing of an artificial organization upon the natural organization of the body. -Thomas Henry Huxley

Time to get way too real. I have friends. Every time we hang out, they are always worried about another dude. What he drives, where he works. Always harping on why some female is with this other dude. Newsflash: Stop being a bitch, man, for real! Stop being a sucker man.

When you develop your skills, when you invest in yourself, you can't really be jealous of other guys. You would recognize that if you had his body, his face, you would still not have the skills you have now. I'd have to work for a long time to master that body. I don't know what type of diseases he has or what type of ailments. He might have sickle-cell anemia, all types of shit you can't see with clothes on. All that stuff affects your stroke, your sex game, affecting your ability to stay focused on the whole process. You don't know about anything except the way that this dude looks. Envy has deep psychological and philosophical roots:

Envy is especially directed at those with whom we compare ourselves, such as our neighbours and relatives. As Bertrand Russell said, 'Beggars do not envy millionaires, though of course they will envy other beggars who are more successful.' Our age of equality and mass media encourages us to compare ourselves to anyone and everyone, fanning the flames of our envy; and by emphasizing the material and tangible over the spiritual and invisible, our culture of empiricism and consumerism has removed the one countervailing force capable of smothering those flames.

The pain of envy is not caused by the desire for the advantages of others per se, but by the feeling of inferiority and frustration occasioned by their lack in ourselves. The distraction of envy and the dread of arousing it in others paradoxically holds us back from achieving our fullest potential. Envy also costs us friends and allies, and, more generally, tempers, restrains, and undermines even our closest relationships. In some cases, it can even lead to acts of sabotage, as with the child who breaks the toy that he knows he cannot have. Over time, our anguish and bitterness can lead to physical health problems such as infections, cardiovascular diseases, and cancers; and mental health problems such as depression, anxiety, and insomnia. We are, quite literally, consumed by envy.[17]

Why would I want to be him when I can be me? When I can look in the mirror and appreciate everything that I bring to the table. Yeah, I know my faults, but you best believe I know the hell out of my strengths. I know how to stroke. I can damn near put a woman through a religious experience using the body I have. Why would I want to be another dude? Why? If I translated my mind into somebody else's form, could I master their abilities like I've mastered my own? No. I couldn't. I would suck if I was them – at the very least, for a good long while. I'm the best at being me, so I'm going to go ahead and be me. I don't know what you're going to do. You can keep on living your life trying to be another person. You can keep on living your life wishing you had somebody else's form and existence. Not me. I'm going to make the best out of what I have. That's what I've been doing ever since I was born. Using what I have to get what I want. Why would I switch now when I'm a master at me? All true practitioners of Stroke Skills come to this realization soon enough.

I think the problem is a lot of you are afraid to even conceive the reality that awaits you once you've claimed the skill set inside of yourself, and that's because you don't practice. You put more investment in everything in your life except believing in yourself, except believing in that body that you have. You put lots of time into school, that new promotion, the money, the car. How can your whole shit be setup just

---

17 https://www.psychologytoday.com/blog/hide-and-seek/201408/the-psychology-and-philosophy-envy

to get her in bed, just to be mediocre when you get her there? And you know it, so the result is you watching her eyes the entire night as she looks at other guys. How lame is that shit? How weak is that?

They said you can't lead a horse, but I'm going to try to lead your ass. I'm going to give you a skill right now, that if you practice it, you're going to ramp your capacity in bed. And on top of that, you're going to have a greater appreciation for your body. You ever seen a boxer throw a right hand? And I know a lot of you don't watch boxing except for the big fights like Paquiao versus Mayweather (because your groupies and your friend had it on). Seriously, do you know anything about boxing? If you don't, I don't care because I'm going to put you on game right now. When you throw a right hand, the boxer isn't hitting his opponent with his right hand. He's hitting his opponent with his legs. Your right hand, your whole body turns into it. The boxer's able to trigger and focus his entire body weight through his two first knuckles into your jaw. That's what happens when you see a boxer through a power right hand. But what if I told you that you can do that with anything that extends off your body? What if I told you that you could do that same thing with your cock? What if I told you, you could put your entire body weight through your cock? Yeah. You think you've put in work; you haven't done shit. You haven't even scratched the surface.

A lot of you try to convince yourself that you already know what I'm telling you. In reality, you don't. You don't know anything about inflating a spot and popping it. You don't know anything about how to work walls based upon the way she moves her body. You don't know how to read a woman like that. You guys are having orgasms with chicks because you're lucky.

A certain number of you out there are like Lebron James, just naturally (or hopefully) gifted. I can give that to you. You came out of the womb just knowing how to work it out. But you're not doing it with any intelligence. You understand? That means you can't do repeat actions. You're not going to be able to know how to stroke one woman versus another based upon how they are built, based upon the way that they shaped, based upon how they move. Nah, you're going to do the same thing with every chick.

Now before you all say, "nah, that ain't me, that ain't me," let me tell you first. I don't care. I don't care what you want. I'm going to put your ignorant ass on game anyway. This is how you throw a power stroke. I told you, when Mayweather throws that power right hand, he puts his whole body behind it. You're not getting hit with his arms, you're not getting hit with his fists, you're getting hit with his neck, his back, and his shoulders. You're getting hit with both legs, both feet and his hips. Everything is punching you in the face when he does that. And like I said, you can do the exact same thing with anything through any appendage. So you'll see guys like Ernesto Hoist, if you guys know anything about kickboxing, you'll see this guy throw kicks and he can kick straight through your leg. He kicks through cinder blocks with his shin, and that's because he's not kicking with just his legs. He's kicking with his neck, his back, his torso. He's kicking with his hips and his chest. It's the exact same thing with your cock.

Here's a secret: any time you watch a video of someone throwing a power shot, whether it's a roundhouse kick, whether it's a straight right, whether it's Tyson throwing a loop then right or a power uppercut, I want you to study their mechanics. All of them. Even baseball players when they're cracking a home run. They sit into their shit. They sit into the punch; they sit into the kick. They'll sit into the power swing. All of them do it because what it does is centralize and localize power at that one place, at that one appendage. An appendage (for you jokers out there that don't have any vocabulary) is an arm or some type of thing extending from your body. So, your arms, your legs, your cock – they're all appendages, you understand?

Back to the point, sit into your stroke. When you stroke, it's not about just pushing with your hips or pushing with your legs. That's not what it's about. What you're going to do is align yourself with her chocha, align yourself with her vaginal opening and then you're going to ground yourself and you're going to use the back of your heels to push your whole form forward. And when you do it, you're going to lift off of one foot. What this is going to do is load all of your weight onto one leg so that when you push those hips forward, your whole body weight is going to go into the stroke. That right there is the hardest stoke that you can throw. But throw at something; what do you know about targeting? What do you know about angling? What do you know about the 80/10/10? What do you know about what strokes are supposed to be doing inside of her? If you don't have this information, you're going to be throwing some really hard strokes at dead space, bro.

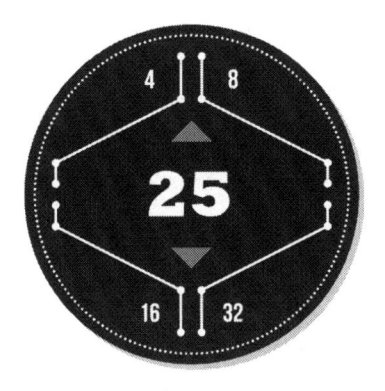

REVERBERATION STROKING

Today a young man on Acid realized that all matter is merely energy condensed to a slow vibration. - Unknown

During sex, touch is vital. Contact is not only very sensual, it is the building block of pleasure. One of the main issues with sex as portrayed in the media is that there is so little contact. The woman usually stays in one position and then the man just jackhammers into her. This rapid fire and single position, especially in the beginning of the exchange, may look good on film, but it is not sensual nor is it enjoyable for women. It should also have considerably more contact than just a quick in an out motion and two people touching at the hips only.

So often, the sensual side of sex is limited to external touching; using the fingers, hands and the tongue to tease an orgasm from your partner by caressing the outside of her body. We know how to touch, where to touch, how light or how hard to caress the clitoris to get your partner to orgasm but so often, it ends there. The attention to touch, pressure and motion ends there and sex itself is almost more of an encore for her, often one without orgasm. Enter the reverberation concept.

Reverberation stroking is all about the science of touch and the transfer of energy that a simple touch can have. Using this technique, you can reach those hard to reach pleasure zones by moving in such a way that causes a transfer of energy from where you are touching her, to other parts of her body. This will open up waves of pleasure, adding to and enhancing the orgasm experience.

To understand what reverberation stroking is and how you can incorporate it into the bedroom, it helps to experience a little bit of the principle yourself. Reverberation stroking is based on energetic sensory relay. Energetic sensory relay is created when you use motion to build up and help transfer energy from one part of the body to another. Consider our bodies: our skin and muscles contain many sensors and nerves. We are very sensitive to touch and energetic sensory relay involves those sensors and nerves because it is possible to use touch in one spot on the body, to transfer across the closest sensors and nerves that touch energy to another part of the body.

Here is an example. Use a finger and push down on the skin on your arm, rubbing a spot on your skin until you feel the skin become heated and warm with the energy that you are creating by rubbing it. Now, without lifting your finger, drag your finger across your skin and then lift up your finger. You will feel the sensation of touch on your skin as if your finger is still dragging along your skin; that is the built up energy that you created that continues in the same direction that you told the energy to go, after lifting up your finger.

Now, consider the vaginal walls. The vaginal walls contain even more sensors and nerve endings than your arm. The vaginal walls are some of the most sensitive areas on the body and that allows you to use reverberation stroking to do what you just did on your arm, on the most sensual and pleasurable areas that she has. You can use your body to build up the energy and then direct it into her body, through her vaginal walls.

The purpose of this is to allow you to stimulate the deeper sensual zones in her body. Many women like the sensation of having their deeper vaginal erogenous zones stimulated, but deep penetrations, deep enough to fully hit the zones inside her vaginal walls can be uncomfortable, especially if the sensors are weak. Deep penetration can also cause dryness, which is certainly not pleasurable.

Reverberation strokes are good for hitting deep spots, where penetration that deep might hurt, or areas that might not be shallow. Not all women have sensors that are shallow, located just behind the vaginal walls. Some women might have sensors that might require more pressure on the vaginal walls, due to having thicker vaginal walls. Putting pressure that is too hard on the vaginal walls can be painful, but you can use reverberation stroking to put pressure where you need to on the vaginal walls and then use the principle of energetic sensory relay to send the motion to where the sensor lies, stimulating them.

You can stay shallow within her sensitive areas, and then use a reverberation stroke to build up that energy and then send it towards her arousal sensors. Reverberation strokes are like revving a car: you rev the engine, and then you lift your foot off the pedal and the car goes. With reverberation strokes, what moves is the transfer of energy into the deep recesses of her body, allowing you to stimulate the harder to reach areas easily.

To build up the energy, you apply the pressure that you want just over the right spot and you go back and forth, just like you did on your arm. Focus your touch on one small area and then you release the stroke, moving deeper in her, keeping your stroke so that the pressure from your stroke is still on the vaginal wall you are targeting. When you move forward, to release the stroke that built up energy will race through her sensors and nerve endings, moving from the spot you were touching, right where you want it to go.

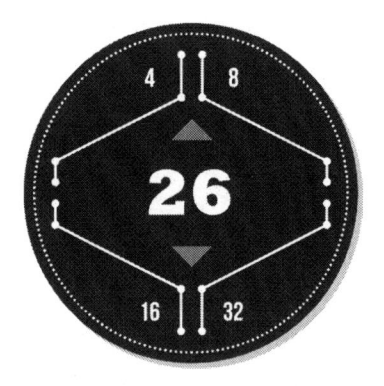

WOMEN THAT ARE SHOOK ABOUT CONFIDENCE

The more they rub, the more you will shine. That Brilliance is yours, and can never be taken from you. - Marrett Green

I'm going to speak to you about a reality that you're going to come into contact through your investment in training your sexual physique and investing in your sexual self-worth. You have to understand that a lot of people can't tell the difference between arrogance and feeling good about who you are and what you're doing. Many of the women that you've dealt with in the past are going to treat you differently when they see you again after you've begun your training. Now some, are going to be really nice. Some are going to be accommodating and proud of you, but unfortunately, a vast majority is going to feel as though you are being arrogant, because your attitude has changed. They're going to pick up on it.

They can read you. So, you might not even say anything. It's not like you're going to be in front of her talking about your skills. You're not going to go into that with her. But, she will sense something is different about you. When she speaks to you now, you're not killing yourself to get and keep her attention. You don't divert your plans suddenly to 'puppy dog' after her and whatever she's doing. It may be difficult to recognize and correct this behavior, because romantic movies and music today have this same message (either overtly or covertly): you're a man, so you're naturally a mess, blessed to simply even stand next to her. Those days of putting women on pedestals simply for breathing are done. Relationship coach Corey Wayne shares what is always the result of this corrosive "pleaser" epidemic:

Women like men who act like men. Men who act more like a man than the woman they are dating. When a man tries to change who he is in order to become what he thinks he needs to become in order to attract the woman he desires, all he does is causes the woman to lose respect for him, because he is not acting like a man. A woman likes a man who makes choices that will make himself happy, instead of making himself miserable by bending himself into a pretzel in order to gain the favor or approval of a woman. Men who do this are acting like a little boy who is seeking the approval of his mommy. Women can't love men they have no respect for and will fall out of love with a man if they lose respect for him over time due to weak pleaser behavior. Relationships are about dating an equal, not taking care of someone who can't or won't take care of themselves, fixing someone or trying to make an imperfect person into the perfect person by changing them or acting like a parent to them.[18]

When she speaks to you now, you're not really concerned about sex with her. You speak about what your ambitions are, what you're doing in life, how you're making things happen, and how lucky some woman is going to be when they finally get a load of you. When you start acting and behaving like that, you give off a different type of energy. You give off an attractive energy. Let me explain that.

When you give off this type of energy, it makes people start saying "what the fuck is he on? What is he thinking about? What is going on in his mind?" And that's the kind of thing that is catnip to women. I can promise you. They want to figure you out. And when you attain this internal peace within yourself, you're going to be a lot harder to discern. More of a challenge. Is that clear?

Some of them are going to try to bring you down because of this. Some of them will try to throw you off of your game. You have to realize that it's not your problem. It's not your problem that they are uncomfortable with your change. You have to let them deal with that. And when this happens, instead of getting mad about it, instead of lashing out, instead of thinking about how come the world isn't on your side and why nobody appreciates you, just realize that it's working. That's it. Realize that people can see it, smell it, feel it. In a world of desperate guys constantly looking for approval from women to feel good about their sexuality, you stand apart because you know

---

18   https://understandingrelationships.com/men-who-are-pleasers/16447

(already going in) that you are one of the best in the world simply because you train.

Now, you go in with a strategy. I know exactly what I'm going to do to this woman, and if, if she really makes me feel good, I might take it to the next level, but I'm not sure about that. You can actually gauge the intensity of sex that you can give a woman based upon the way you're feeling about her and her reciprocity. See, that's a different type of mindset. It's one that puts you in the alpha position. It's one that puts you in control of the situation. You recognize that you are the gem. You recognize that you are the gift and you recognize that your strokes are a blessing. You become fire. Many fear being burned by you, yet crave warmth from the essential heat only a man like you can provide.

> Emaun Wilson » Stroke Skills ELITE
> 1 hr · Edited
>
> My fiancée hit me with a drop stroke move, when I wasn't expecting it last night. Now my head is all messed up, and I'm in my feelings. Good thing we are engaged, or I might have to stalk him! Smh
>
> Unlike · Comment

James recognized The Gotan Project's European synth-flair and hypnotic beat as he came off the elevator to the third floor of the storage facility. It played from a portable radio to his left. He wanted to give props to the woman standing in the middle of the hallway in that indoor storage facility. The music came from some portable stereo of hers. He wanted to, but he stopped himself. Her frizzy, auburn tinged hair was in two ponytails, a hairstyle much too immature for such an agitated twenty-something. But then there were the tattoos... Japanese fishes, Sanskrit sayings and cockatoo birds that made colorful sleeves out of her toned and bare arms that somewhat justified the hair – and the snug cut-off jeans. As soon as he saw a glimpse of her seasoned quads between the waist-high U-Haul boxes that surrounded her, he knew she would have been just the type of woman he would have been a straight up bitch for.

A few months back.

He knew the old James would have instantly wished to not have come from the house in Adidas sandals, V-neck T-shirt and Dickies work pants. He would have belittled his lean frame by hunching his shoulders over and a scratched his long neck to apologize for needing to get by. He would have gushed over her taste in music, interviewed her as to where she first learned of the group... she would be put off by his eagerness, as they always did, which prompt him to crack a lame joke to keep from completely turning her off. James grinned. Ha! That was him, just a month or so ago. That pool-stick stroking loser.

The woman, unaware of him, wiped her face and walked into her opened unit. Instead of tripping over the boxes to introduce himself as he would have done, he strolled by with hands in his camo short's pockets, or at least tried to stroll by, until the boxes kept him from making it on by to his own storage unit. He cleared his throat and looked about as if to say, glad I ain't the one to get this straightened out.

The woman sighed. James looked up at her as if surprised a human came with the boxes. She had to be mixed for those freckles, he thought. Standing between an old Lazy Boy, two matching cranberry couches and opened boxes of shoes and clothes, she scratched through her Wonder Woman T-shirt to the center of her flat chest. Her coffee brown eyes held no expression. "What, you gotta get by?" She looked around, closed her eyes and exhaled. "Look, I'm sorry." She raised her hand up. "Just, hold on."

James nodded to the Gotan Project's *Diferente* and slowly bent over to move a box. "Yeah well, let me –"

The woman came closer, her tiny fingers splayed out as if stopping a car for backing up. "Just, please –okay?"

James shrugged his shoulders and stood up. "I'm standing right here, lady." James put his big hands out, not as if let her inspect his palms, more like he was cupping a woman's ass. "Got two good hands."

The woman stammered. Her eyes darted from his hands to his eyes and back, "No. No it's perfectly fine."

James put his hands down. The woman started shoving a box out of his way.

"What's your name?"

The woman exhaled as she finished moving the box aside. "Are you really – " she scratched at her left ear. He could tell she was about to look down at something on him but caught herself. She exhaled, as if what she was about to do was a bad idea. "Mya." She shoved an opened box of coats to the side.

James walked away. No, 'gee that's a pretty name, what does it mean?' crap. No attempt to press for more info. No creepy questions to see if she was really there at 10 o'clock at night, by herself moving things around. Or if she had a boyfriend. No. He left it as just enough small talk to talk until she got her shit out of the way for him to pass.

James pulled his pea coat, three quarter trench coat, and sweaters out of a box for the coming months and lay them on a cart out in the hallway. He nodded to the music and delighted in hearing Mya down the hall shifting boxes and fussing with someone over her cell phone. He smirked and licked his lips. Sucks to be her.

The former club DJ noticed an old mixing board over by the ramps he bought in order to change the oil on his Mazda. His very first mixing board, a Numark Mixtrack. He wiped sweat from his face. Those were the days; experimenting with house music and underground hip hop in his mother's basement.

"Umm."

James looked to the hallway. Mya stood at the opening with her arms folded and mouth twisted. She looked off to the side as if refusing to meet James' eyes. James gathered his things, deciding not to address her as of yet.

Mya exhaled. "Excuse me."

James turned back to her slowly.

Mya's eyes met his for a brief moment before she tilted her head to the side and scratched at an eyebrow. "There's another box you could help with if you want."

James pointed at his chest. Me? Mya rolled her eyes.

"I don't know. You seem to be a lil' put off by my presence."

"Look, you know, a lot is going on. I'm just – "

James came out of the unit his forearms glistening with sweat. He closed his unit door and looked into her eyes. Like a man pouring water into a vessel. Her opened mouth went still.

"Whatever your deal is, I think you can do better though."

Mya began to stammer again.

"For me, you can do better."

Mya closed her eyes. "Fine. Ok."

Her reply fell onto his ears softer than her flustered haze. To a sweetness, one that could not be that foreign to her.

Mya slowly nodded and made a sarcastic bow with a motion to direct him to her unit.

He leaned back against his unit's opened door. I ain't playing with you.

Mya's face relaxed. Finally! "Ok, I'm sorry. What's your name?"

"James." Now his own voice fell to a more comforting tone.

The stroll to her unit felt surreal, like getting her number was inevitable. It was if he had walked into a movie, with her stereo playing the soundtrack. Mya sighed and pointed to four heavy boxes by her unit door. "I need those in the back corner on top of each other, please."

James made a point of getting it done with no help from her, bending his knees and getting them in one after the other. Mya bent over this coffee table and that couch, ass high up in the air, to make room for him. He obliged, bumping into her enough to smell the slight dampness of perspiration. More than once. Or was she bumping into him? Oh yes, the new confidence drew it out of her.

She leaned into him from behind, putting her slightly hardening nipple against his back. "Yeah, right there is good."

James looked back at her.

Mya licked her thick pink, bare lips. "Sorry. I'm a lil wet. Wait! I mean -"

"Say no more."

She laughed nervously.

Yes, she was definitely bumping into him. Her voice became more throaty and accommodating with every box. And so, after the second box, he asked about her origin and let the exchange flow organically to sharing that he was a DJ. Organically.

Mya explained that she was a tattoo artist moving out of an apartment with a now former fiancé.

James thought of the progression of strokes he would use on her. He nodded and brushed past her for the third box. "Oh, that's what that frustration was all about. Sorry to hear that."

Mya smiled. Yeah, right.

The stereo, a little Dre Beats pill, shifted to an extended dance track by Fat Freddy. James noticed Mya going down the hall as he shifted the third box against the wall. She returned as he strolled up to the last box.

"There isn't another cart around beside the one you have, James?"

James bent down to the box to hide how rapturous it was to hear her say his name. "Doubt it, Mya. I'll bring it back up when I'm done." He smiled. There was nothing left outside of her unit to put on a cart. His skin began to tingle.

When he finished with the box, Mya sat on his cart, her thighs wide enough to make her look like she needed to be smoking a cigarette. "So, guess that's it."

James came to her. On the verge of a full on erection, he took her by the hand to help her up from the cart. He caught her sneaking a look at his crotch. Kissing her on her forehead, he led her into the unit. He felt her lean into him again, clutching at his arm, trusting his lead, her nose into his shoulder blade, taking in his scent.

"Thank you. I mean, you know what I mean."

James turned around and kissed her forehead again. Then her lips. Yes, he did know. In a way that would have never let him trust his instincts enough to know before. Had he truly become his own super hero? Was a little confidence in the mechanics of sex all it took? Looking to find out, he caught her when she swayed, feeling her mind's vibration: Oh shit, here I go. Yes, he said in his own vibration: Absolutely.

"I'm sticky. I'm sweaty."

James slipped a middle finger along the small of her damp back to wrap the waist band of her thong around it. Guiding her hips to the darkness of the boxes in the corner by the thong's band like a ring in a bull's nose. Stepping over a handi-vac and a pile of books and positioned himself behind her. He kissed her soft, cool and slightly salty neck. She placed her hands on the boxes.

"I don't even fucking know you." she whispered, to herself it seemed. "Somebody might come."

James cupped her sex. "Somebody deserves to."

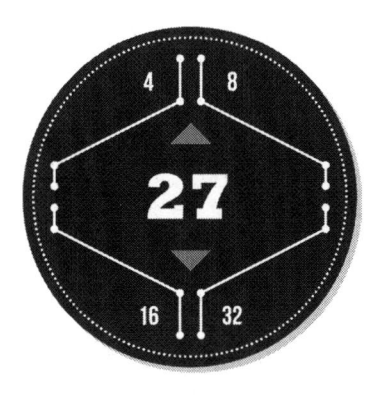

LACK OF CONSISTENCY

Trust is built with consistency. - Lincoln Chafee

There is nothing wrong with wanting to win. There is nothing wrong with wanting respect. There is nothing wrong with wanting to feel wanted and feel understood, to feel like someone believes in you and feel like someone has your back. These are vital aspects of being a man. You need these things to be able to build into yourself and although you want such validation from other people, you want know it and enjoy it within yourself most of all.

We're in time right now where external validation has people living inside out for Facebook likes. Things are changing so fast around us is it's hard to be able to hold onto anything for balance and context. It's hard to be able to find out what is real and truly gratifying, so we find ourselves bouncing from job to job, from opportunity to opportunity and even from woman to woman.

Let's say, for right now, the woman you're with right now could be that cheerleader for you and root for you as you strive to be your best? What if you can change things so that she no longer questions everything that you say? What if things went back to the point where you can look at her and know that she believed in you, in your potential– what if you can go back to that? It's possible, but you have to understand how she got that way. You have to understand that it's not her fault, she's human. You can't just look at the end result and think that you played no part in it because in doing that, you cancel your own capacity to change. If you steal your own ability to reflect on how you got to where you are and what role you played in it, you're damned to consistently repeat the same problems over and over again.

So how does that relate and respond to her? Have you ever asked her how many things she was excited about that you said you were going to do and just didn't do? Ever asked yourself how the things she dreamt of and how joyous she was when you told her this was something that you were going to participate in and then you swept it off the table?

You can look at her engaging you the way that she is now as her protecting her own essence. Our essence is developed from faith in dreams sustained and realized as well as situations where faith in dreams are dashed and thrown away. This can change who we are as a people. Maybe, just maybe, she wants to be able to hold onto a part of herself that still loves you. Maybe she puts up that barrier so you can't see how injured she is that things turned out differently.

Most of us haven't because as men in this world hunting, fighting and killing what we have to eat every day, we can't afford to look at everyone else's feelings because we know that if we miss a step, the whole board falls. When the king falls, the game is over– but at the same time, your queen is a person that can recharge you. She can build into you and make you something better, help you recognize the realness that's inside of you. However, she will not be satiated if you are not maintaining the relationship. That queen will turn cold to protect herself. In a world that makes conflict sexier than harmony, it may require counseling to discover how communication is not a contest, but a collaboration:

One of the biggest problems in communicating is that most couples have a basic misconception of what the purpose of communication is. Most approach talking with a partner as a debate in which each presents a preconceived version of the reality of what is going on between the two partners. The fault with this approach is the mistaken assumption that either partner can go into the conversation with an accurate perception of reality. This is not possible because neither person has the necessary information to determine what reality is, that is: what is going on between them. One purpose of communication is to determine what reality is. Communication involves the collaboration of two people as they share and examine all of their perceptions, feelings, ideas and thoughts to come to an accurate understanding of what is happening.[19]

After you've put in the time and effort, ultimately you must realize that

---

19 http://www.psychalive.org/communication-between-couples/

there is nothing that you can change about someone else. There is only your capacity to change *yourself,* so what responsibility and action do you take for being inconsistent and inconsiderate of dreams and aspirations you have foiled because of what you had to do to survive? How do you do to remedy that? The answer is finding something and remaining consistent. I was able to invest in my capacity to please my woman. Each and every time I was with her, I was able to reinforce the notion that no matter what happens on this external plane, no matter what opportunities I leave on the table and which opportunities I take, no matter which partnerships, no matter which deals rise and fall from day-to-day, do not mistake that I do not have you in my mind and heart.

I make her understand this which each and every stroke, help her to recognize this with each and every orgasm. Every time she came I read that to her. I read into who she was and it changed everything because those enzymes, that serotonin, that dopamine that hit her brain reinforced what I said. It helped her to recognize that just because I have to change to move and shake in the society doesn't mean I'm changing about her. Understand that this woman knew every night when we went into that room that all the bullshit, all the games, the chess moves, the strategy that we as men have to play to survive in this world stayed outside. I was there with her. It was just her and me, together in a way that made nothing else matter.

From that point on when I would tell her about opportunities, when I would tell her about mistakes, when I would tell her about successes, and I would tell her about failures, she would respond the same way:

'you've got this, I know you've got this.' Learning to love a woman is synonymous to fixing your house with solar power. There is no one that can take that energy from you. That is a raw source of empowerment, passion and ambition that will reinforce everything that you want to do, will do and what you dream of doing. There is no more important task than making sure your partner recognizes that no matter what situations arise, she will remain your partner. I urge you to invest in the intimacy and communication skills that will change your life. I urge you today to invest in yourself; invest in stroke skills.

Earl Lane   11:43pm
Whats up Montique... i went ahead and did what you mentioined i stopped complaining about the lack of sex and she and i had a good talk about the other issues we had like money management, etc and i just stareted hitting the weights extra hard no matter what and i incorporated some of the videos i saw from stroke skills. and just said fuck it we may not be having sex now but when we do she will be begging for more... So the other day we made love and well i even surprised myself and now she cant stop thinking about it. so im going to have to get the full program soon because i can only imagine what im not getting by not hvaing th full program.

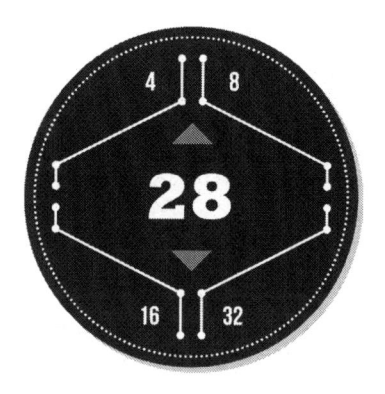

THE BEST FOOD STROKES

Your diet is a bank account; Good food choices are good investments.- Bethenny Frankel

Hey what do you eat before a stroke session? What type of food or nutrition, what type of fuel is best to put inside of your vehicle before you start to stroke? Now a lot of guys like to ingest a lot of alcohol because alcohol allows you to feel less–it numbs you and simultaneously it might drop your inhibitions a little bit; so you might get a little crazier if you drink. But here's the thing, that's for lames. You can't feel her spots if you are numb. I guess the question is, do you want to make her cum or not? You have to be able to feel her rolls; you have to be able to feel her vaginal canal. With that understood, here's more on what heavy drinking does beyond numbness:

Temporary erectile dysfunction. Researchers have found that too much alcohol affects both your brain and your penis. In one University of Washington study, sober men were able to achieve an erection more quickly than intoxicated men — and some men are unable to have an erection at all after drinking.

That's because pre-sex boozing decreases blood flow to your penis, reduces the intensity of your orgasm, and can dampen your level of excitement (in other words, even if you are able to have sex, it may not be nearly as pleasurable as it would be without the excess alcohol).

Long-term erectile dysfunction. The risk for long-term erectile dysfunction has been linked to chronic heavy use of alcohol. In fact, studies show that men who are dependent on alcohol have a 60 to 70 percent chance of suffering from sexual problems. The most common of these are erectile dysfunction, premature ejaculation, and loss of sexual desire.[20]

Back to what you should eat and why. I would not recommend lots of starches, simply because as carbohydrates, they burn out quickly and it's going to take your body energy to burn those carbohydrates. Because the body is using that energy, it's not going to allow you to have extra energy to use in the bedroom. Now given, a lot of you are super human, a lot of you have great genetics, also a lot of you train stroke skills, so you are going to already have an accelerated ability in the bedroom. I am talking about reaching your peak or really being able to deliver your best performance. I wouldn't recommend lots of

---

[20] http://www.everydayhealth.com/erectile-dysfunction/why-boozing-can-be-bad-for-your-sex-life.aspx

starchy carbohydrates like noodles, rice, bread. A lot of these things fill you up; however, you are going to burn out because your body needs to focus a lot of its energy on breaking down these complex carbs. It's going to make you sleepy; that's where the "-itis" comes from.

I recommend green vegetables and water. If you drink water with lime, because lime is citrus, it's alkaline when it hits your body. This is going to allow you to flush a lot of toxins out of your system; it's going to allow your machine to really run. The green vegetables in cells act as fuel, but it's not fuel that is going to make you tired. You are not going to get sleepy after eating these greens. You can eat lots and lots and lots and lots of greens and not get tired. It's not going to put you to sleep like if you eat potatoes, rice, lasagna, or pizza. Even black beans, sad to say, will knock you out at this time when you really want to be the most attentive. Here is more of the foods that will get you more out of your time in bed:

Avocados

The Aztecs referred to avocados as, ahem, testicles, because of their physical shape. But the scientific reason why avocados make sense as an aphrodisiac is that they are rich in unsaturated fats and low in saturated fat, making them good for your heart and your arteries. Anything that keeps the heart beating strong helps keep blood flowing to all the right places. In fact, men with underlying heart disease are twice as likely to suffer from erectile dysfunction (ED).

Almonds

Topping my list of feisty foods, almonds have long been purported to increase passion, act as a sexual stimulant, and aid with fertility. Like asparagus (another one of my favorite sexy foods), almonds are nutrient-dense and rich in several trace minerals that are important for sexual health and reproduction, such as zinc, selenium, and vitamin E. "Zinc helps enhance libido and sexual desire," says Dr. Berman. "We don't really understand the mechanisms behind it, but we know it works."

Strawberries

The color red is known to help stoke the fire: A 2008 study found that men find women sexier if they're wearing red, as opposed to cool colors such as blue or green. Strawberries are also an excellent source of folic acid, a B vitamin that helps ward off birth defects in women and, according to a University of California, Berkley study, may be tied to high sperm counts in men. This Valentine's Day, try making dark-chocolate-dipped strawberries. And while we're on the subject, there's a reason we give chocolate on Valentine's Day: It's full of libido-boosting methylxanthines.

Seafood

Despite their slippery and slimy texture, oysters may be the most well-known aphrodisiac. They're also one of the best sources of libido-boosting zinc. But other types of seafood can also act as aphrodisiacs. Oily fish—like wild salmon and herring—contain Omega 3's which are essential for a healthy heart.

Arugula

Arugula has been heralded as an arousal aid since the first century. Today, research reveals that the trace minerals and antioxidants packed into dark, leafy greens are essential for our sexual health because they help block absorption of some of the environmental contaminants thought to negatively impact our libido.

Figs

These funny-shaped fruits have a long history of being a fertility booster, and they make an excellent aphrodisiac because they are packed with both soluble and insoluble fiber, which is important for heart health. Plus, high-fiber foods help fill you up, not out, so it's easier to achieve that sexy bottom line—or belly.

Citrus

Any member of this tropical fruit family is super-rich in antioxidants, vitamin C, and folic acid—all of which are essential for men's reproductive health. Enjoy a romantic salad that incorporates citrus, like pink grapefruit or mandarin oranges, or use a dressing made with lemon and lime.[21]

Again we have to get out of this whole framework, out of this fuzzy inebriated love making mindset. And a lot of times we are inebriated either from alcohol, from weed or from doing things like eating the wrong stuff before we make love. You want to have your machine running clean. Pay keen attention to this woman's

---

21 http://www.health.com/health/gallery/0,,20307213,00.html

body, to her 'tells' – you want to be able to look at her hands, her feet, notice what she is clinching on. Be able to feel each and every part of her body reacting to you, so that you know how to react to her. When it comes to intimacy and love- making, training like the champion you're born to be requires that you eat like one as well.

CONCLUSION : WHAT WILL YOU LEAVE HERE?

We may give without loving, but we cannot love without giving. - Bernard Meltzer

The big question is: what do we leave on this planet as men? What can we leave here as an imprint that we were here and made a difference? What can we do to ensure that those who come after us can live in a world better than the one that we did? A lot of us might think that it's money. A lot of us might think that it's investments in stocks and bonds— but you have to remember that all those things are man-made and depend on an artificial rule of law which depends on a sequence of future actions to make those things relevant. Invest in what stands as powerful regardless of such fluctuations.

There is something that we can leave here that will stand on its own regardless of how this and that will change. That is a code of conduct that we will be remembered by afterwards. It will draw others to us and we can then enlighten them on this unique way to develop their self-worth. We would actually be reshaping into one where men would not need to persecute others in order to feel powerful. Each of us would feel powerful in and of ourselves; become part of a new archetype in society that revolve around sharing instead of competing.

The only reason that we as men find the need for secrecy and for scarcity is because we don't recognize that we have endless value. Operating from a sense of lack is a ploy used to withhold information so that the information maintains value. It makes us appear better than somebody else, but that's something that men do out of fear. You know you are the best and you know you have these talents and skills that are only inside of *you*. They are connected to the man that you are. You don't have to worry that someone is going to take those things from you. This is not some Utopian society; this is something that you create within the small circle of friends that you have right now. If each of us did this with just the males that we have within our very own circle, we could slowly bring them together – so that we become better men being better for ourselves, our children and the women in our lives.

Invest in yourself. Look deeply into who you are and ask, 'what unique things does this body and this mind offer to a woman?' I want you to look at yourself as a library with several different catalogs and deep, deep trenches filled with information. Fill those trenches with as much knowledge as you can so that you have an ability to use your catalog index to do anything that you need to be able to do. This includes satisfying any woman who would be lucky enough to come across your path and earn your favor.

S.T.R.O.K.E

Bainrigh Robin Cordrey ▸ Stroke Skills ELITE
January 9

What happens when you give a man who already has an amazing bedroom game a few of the SSE secrets?

You get your ass KOed by Stroke Skills!

Yeah that's right, I got myself knocked out! Words cannot begin to describe the overwhelming feelings that a man using SSE can invoke. I am lucky to be speaking in sentences today, and not in some mythical tongue.

He knew exactly what he was doing. (I'm sure it was planned out.) Yet, I had no clue what I was in for. He set the music, engaged the senses, and damn it if he didn't start stroking at the 80! Ladies you know they are always looking to dive in...but NO, he stayed and worked every angle of that 80 until I was begging for more. (good thing he could read body language, cuz I couldn't form a word if I tried) It felt so intoxicating, but I didn't realize exactly what was happening until he told me, in his Alpha voice, to watch us in the mirror, as he was stroking. (UStroke, walk it out, and scrapes) My mind went in spirals. I couldn't believe what I was seeing, while waves of euphoria and bliss washed through my body as his body was moving to the rhythm of the music. The internal yoni massage, that hit spots I never knew existed and the orgasms that erupted...no words will ever be powerful enough to describe them. Then he tells me, "I want you to SEE what you are feeling." (and kept telling we to watch...which was the hardest thing to do since my eyeballs were rolling up into my head in true Exorcist fashion) Right there! That connection of SEEING those moves I've seen videos of several times being USED on me...I died and went to heaven. All I can say is I WANT MORE!

Montique, get those SSE cards ready, cuz I guarantee that once women experience this for themselves they won't ever want to be intimate with a man again unless he has one.

%?F www.faceb...

William's arms shook and burned post-orgasm as he lowered himself, in the darkness, down into Destiny's frantic embrace around his neck. A passing car's headlights brushed across the room from the window. She had lifted herself up to crush her chest against his still-racing heart. Pulling him down onto the bed as she still convulsed. Whispering it into the side of his neck again: So fuckin' proud of you.

William wiped the sweat from his twitching face by smearing it into the down-feathered pillow Destiny lay her head on. He exhaled deeply as her screams still echoed in his mind. She had never lost herself in the moment like that before. There was no argument beforehand to set up the frantic intensity of making up. He closed his eyes and let them roll under his eyelids from the thought of simply catching her by surprise with his new skills. Of solving some sarcastic and impatient riddle deep inside her in a way that made her squeal and gasp with its level of precision. William and this man's work of his had given birth to something. He knew it. Something Destiny would never be forget. That love song by Foreigner that his uncle used to play, "I Wanna Know What Love Is," that and any other one with that same stadium anthem feel to it, suddenly made sense.

Destiny sighed and laughed nervously. Then sniffled. He could just faintly smell her underarms. Oh yes, she had lost her cool this time. He could feel her trying to retreat back to where they were hours before... before the sweet tease of the 80-10-10, the unparalleled oral that had her turning it into a 69 only to be thrown off her task from the orgasm he gave her, the Latin merengue from the inverted missionary position, the lift and drop combos and plank scrapes after flipping her over that he had practiced for three weeks while she was out of town.

William replayed how Destiny stopped him, trying to figure it out as she pushed him back with trembling legs. He grinned at being smart and staying close enough to base stroke through it. He could feel the heat of her looking into his eyes in the dark. He had never felt before the confidence, the understanding of sexual geometry. William never knew this feeling before. When he was as common as the next man and was treated as such. He lifted up to see what he could of her features in the dark. Destiny held him around his neck like they were slow dancing. She whispered what sounded like a prayer and then, in spite of her fear, said it again. So fuckin' proud of you. He lowered himself turned onto his back. She lay her head on his chest.

William could feel her brain going warm with thoughts. Where did he get that from? How am I going to deal with this? He kissed her sweaty forehead and felt wrinkles. Her eyebrows had to be high up over her eyes. An expression of wonder? She shifted her features against his neck. He felt the smooth enamel of her front teeth on his chest. Smiling, perhaps? Still erect enough from his orgasm, mostly due to this new plateau, he thought of getting on top of her into an easy base stroke. He let the thought pass when it was clear that she was on the verge of sobbing. From joy.

He longed for the side of a mountain to stand, like a lion over his pride and overlook what was now his; this new vision for his life and any woman willing to hold tight to have his wisdom, time and care imbued into her being.

Made in the USA
Charleston, SC
21 September 2016